D1565063

Nicotine Safety and Toxicity

Nicotine Safety and Toxicity

edited by
Neal L. Benowitz, M.D.

New York   Oxford
Oxford University Press
1998

Oxford University Press

Athens   Auckland   Bangkok   Bogota   Bombay
Buenos Aires   Calcutta   Cape Town   Dar es Salaam
Delhi   Florence   Hong Kong   Istanbul   Karachi
Kuala Lumpur   Madras   Madrid   Melbourne
Mexico City   Nairobi   Paris   Singapore
Taipei   Tokyo   Toronto   Warsaw

and associated companies in
Berlin   Ibadan

Copyright © 1998 by Oxford University Press

Published by Oxford University Press, Inc.
198 Madison Avenue, New York, New York 10016

Library of Congress Cataloging-in-Publication Data
Nicotine safety and toxicity / edited by Neal L. Benowitz.
p.   cm. Includes bibliographical references and index.
ISBN 0-19-511496-5
1. Nicotine—Toxicology—Congresses.
2. Nicotine—Therapeutic use—Evaluation—Congresses.
I. Benowitz, Neal L.
II. Society for Research on Nicotine and Tobacco.
[DNLM: 1. Nicotine—toxicity—congresses.   QV   137   N6623   1998]
RA1242.N5N55   1998
616.86'5—dc21
DNLM/DLC
for Library of Congress   97-46155

1 2 3 4 5 6 7 8 9

Printed in the United States of America
on acid-free paper

PREFACE

Nicotine has long been considered one of the toxic chemicals in tobacco that contributes to tobacco-related disease. It is certainly toxic to insects and is widely used as an insecticide in household products such as Black Leaf 40 (40% nicotine sulfate). In high doses, nicotine is toxic to people. There have been numerous reports of accidental, and some of intentional, human intoxications or deaths.* The toxic effects of nicotine from tobacco have been exploited by South American shamans during ritual ceremonies involving death-like states from which the shaman miraculously recovers, thereby reinforcing the appearance of his supernatural powers.†

Importantly, nicotine in tobacco maintains nicotine addiction, the proximate cause of tobacco-related disease, which claims millions of lives each year throughout the world. Whether the nicotine in tobacco is directly toxic to body organs is unclear.

Nicotine's toxicity is important not only in understanding the effects of tobacco use, but also because nicotine is being developed as a potential medication for diseases other than tobacco addiction. Nicotine acts on nicotinic cholinergic receptors in the brain and elsewhere. These receptors have numerous and complex effects on psychological, neurohormonal, cardiovascular, and other physiological processes.‡ Some of the diseases for which nicotine is being considered as a therapeutic agent are ulcerative colitis, Alzheimer's disease, Parkinson's disease, Tourette syndrome, dystonia, sleep apnea, abscess ulcers, attention deficit disorder, obesity, and chronic inflammatory skin disorders. Of these, the clinical investigation of nicotine is actively ongoing for the treatment of ulcerative colitis, Alzheimer's disease, and Parkinson's disease.

The feasibility of using a drug like nicotine, for which there are concerns about toxicity, depends on the balance of benefits versus risks. Benefits are now being addressed in clinical trials. The potential risks of nicotine are the subject of this book.

To address the safety and toxicity of nicotine, a group of experts met on De-

*Beeman JA, Hunter WC: Fatal nicotine poisoning. A report of twenty-four cases. *Archives of Pathology* 1937, 24:481–485.

†Wilbert J: *Tobacco and Shamanism in South America.* New Haven: Yale University Press, 1987.

‡Benowitz NL: Pharmacology of nicotine: Addiction and therapeutics. *Annual Review of Pharmacology and Toxicology* 1996, 36:597–613.

cember 6, 1996, in Braselton, Georgia. At a symposium entitled "The Safety and Toxicity of Nicotine," sponsored by the Society for Research on Nicotine and Tobacco, they examined basic and clinical data on the pharmacology and toxicology of nicotine. This information was considered in the context of the pathophysiology of tobacco-related diseases to assess the potential risks of nicotine, per se, in humans. The symposium concluded with the experts appraising the risks of nicotine to humans, assigning different levels of probability, and identifying areas for future research. Papers presented at this meeting are the basis for the chapters in this book, which reviews the current understanding of the safety and toxicity of nicotine.

San Francisco, Calif.   N.L.B.
November 1997

CONTENTS

CONTRIBUTORS

Raymond J. Alderfer, M.D., M.P.H.
Center for Drug Evaluation and Research
Food and Drug Administration
Rockville, MD

Neal L. Benowitz, M.D.
Division of Clinical Pharmacology
Departments of Medicine, Psychiatry
    and Biopharmaceutical Sciences
University of California
San Francisco, CA

Anna Borukhova, M.S.
Chemical Carcinogenesis
American Health Foundation
Valhalla, NY

Steven G. Carmella, B.S.
University of Minnesota Cancer Center
Minneapolis, MN

Kay Castagnoli, B.S.
Department of Chemistry
Virginia Polytechnic Institute and State
    University
Blacksburg, VA

Neal Castagnoli, Jr., Ph.D.
Department of Chemistry
Virginia Polytechnic Institute and State
    University
Blacksburg, VA

Kathleen Daniels, M.S.
School of Public Health
University of Minnesota
Minneapolis, MN

David M. Daughton, M.S.
Department of Internal Medicine
Pulmonary and Critical Care Section
University of Nebraska Medical Center
Omaha, NE

Harriet de Wit, Ph.D.
Department of Psychiatry
University of Chicago
Chicago, IL

Chrisoula Eliopoulos, M.Sc.
Division of Clinical Pharmacology and
    Toxicology
Department of Pediatrics
The Hospital for Sick Children
Toronto, Ontario, Canada

Roger A. Goetsch, Pharm.D.
Postmarketing Safety Evaluation Dept.
Center for Drug Evaluation and Research
Food and Drug Administration
Rockville, MD

Steve Gourlay, M.D., MBBS, Ph.D.
Department of Epidemiology
University of California
and Genentech, Inc.
San Francisco, CA

John Green, M.B. Ch.B., MRCP
Gastroenterology
Department of Medicine
University Hospital, Wales
Heathpark
Cardiff, UK

Hildur Hardardottir, M.D.
Maternal Fetal Medicine
Department of Obstetrical Gynecology
University of Connecticut Health Center
Farmington, CT

Stephen S. Hecht, Ph.D.
University of Minnesota Cancer Center
Minneapolis, MN 55455

Jack E. Henningfield, Ph.D.
Pinney Associates, Inc.
Bethesda, MD

Stephen J. Heishman, Ph.D
National Institute On Drug Abuse
Clinical Pharmcology Branch
Baltimore, MD

John Hughes, M.D.
Department of Psychiatry
University of Vermont
Burlington, VT

Julia Klein, M.Sc.
Division of Clinical Pharmacology and
    Toxicology
Department of Pediatrics
The Hospital for Sick Children
Toronto, Ontario, Canada

Gideon Koren, M.D.
Division of Clinical Pharmacology and
    Toxicology
Department of Pediatrics
The Hospital for Sick Children
Toronto, Ontario, Canada

E. Douglas Kramer, M.D.
Medical Review Office
Center for Drug Evaluation and Research
Food and Drug Administration
Rockville, MD

Xin Liu, Ph.D.
Drug Metabolism
3M Pharmaceuticals
St. Paul, MN

Atkinson W. Longmire, M.D.
Medical Review Office
Center for Drug Evaluation and Research
Food and Drug Administration
Rockville, MD

Robert P. Murray, Ph.D.
The Alcohol and Tobacco Research Unit
Department of Community Health
    Sciences and University of Manitoba
Winnipeg, Manitoba, Canada

Cheryl A. Oncken, M.D., MPH
Department of Medicine
University of Connecticut Health Center
Farmington, CT

Stephen I. Rennard, M.D.
Department of Internal Medicine
Pulmonary and Critical Care Section
University of Nebraska Medical Center
Omaha, NE

John Rhodes, M.B. Ch.B., M.D., FRCP
University Hospital, Wales
Heathpark
Cardiff, UK

Hildegard M. Schuller, Ph.D., D.V.M.
Department of Pathobiology
University of Tennessee
College of Veterinary Medicine
Knoxville, TN

Mark K. Shigenaga, Ph.D.
Department of Molecular and Cell Biology
Division of Biochemistry and Molecular
    Biology
University of California, Berkeley
Berkeley, CA

Theodore A. Slotkin, Ph.D.
Department of Pharmacology
Duke University Medical Center
Durham, NC

James S. Smeltzer, M.D.
Maternal Fetal Medicine
Department of Obstetrical Gynecology
University of Connecticut Health Center
Farmington, CT

Daniel A. Spyker, Ph.D., M.D.
Division of Cardiovascular Respiratory
and Neurological Devices
Center for Devices and Radiological
Health
Food and Drug Administration
Rockville, MD

Maxine L. Stitzer, Ph.D.
Department of Psychiatry and Behavioral
Sciences
Johns Hopkins University School of
Medicine
Bayview Medical Center
Baltimore, MD

Goreth A. O. Thomas, MB ChB., M.D., MRCP
Gastroenterology
Department of Medicine
University Hospital, Wales
Heathpark
Cardiff, UK

Richard Wardrop III, B.S.
Department of Medical Microbiology and
Immunology
University of Ohio
Columbus, OH

Ake Wennmalm, M.D., Ph.D.
Goteborg University
Sahlgrenska University Hospital
Goteborg, Sweden

John Windle, M.D.
Department of Internal Medicine
Cardiology Section
University of Nebraska Medical Center
Omaha, NE

Nicotine Safety and Toxicity

Nicotine Pharmacology and Addiction

NEAL L. BENOWITZ

Nicotine, the main determinant of tobacco use and addiction, is now available as a medication to assist smoking cessation and is being evaluated as a medication for a variety of other medical disorders. Although this book focuses on the safety and toxicity of nicotine, Chapter 1 provides an overview of the basic and clinical pharmacology of nicotine and how nicotine contributes to tobacco addiction. The reader is also referred to the 1987 Surgeon General's Report, *The Health Consequences of Smoking: Nicotine Addiction,*[1] and other reviews.[2,3] for a detailed description of the pharmacology of nicotine and its role in tobacco addiction.

Mechanisms of action

Nicotine is a tertiary amine consisting of a pyridine and a pyrrolidine ring (Fig. 1-1). (S)-Nicotine, found in tobacco, binds stereoselectively to nicotinic cholinergic receptors. (R)-Nicotine, found in small quantities in cigarette smoke due to racemization during the pyrolysis process, and commonly used in pharmacological studies, is a weak agonist at cholinergic receptors.

Nicotinic cholinergic receptors are found in the brain and autonomic ganglia, and the neuromuscular nicotinic cholinergic receptor has been well characterized as a ligand-gated ion channel composed of five subunits.[4]

Most relevant to nicotine addiction are the neuronal nicotinic acetylcholine receptors. The receptors are found throughout the brain, with the greatest number of

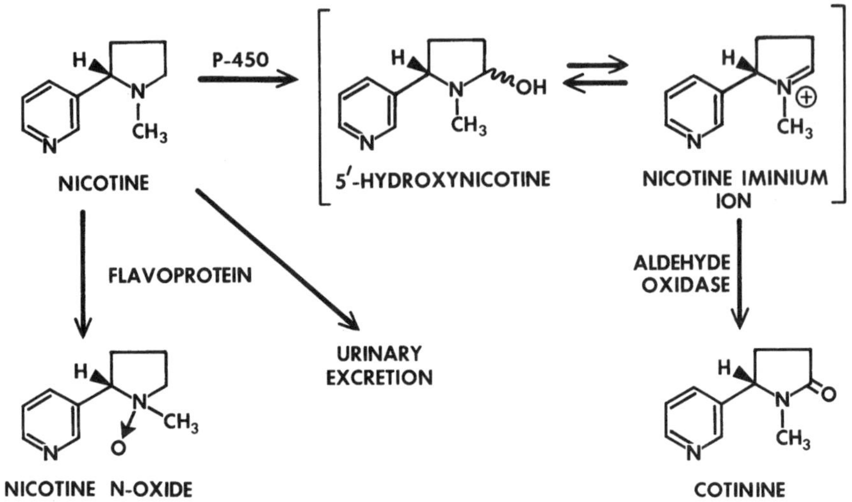

Figure 1-1. Chemical structure of nicotine and major pathways of nicotine metabolism (Reprinted from Benowitz et al.,[27] with permission of the publisher.)

binding sites in the cortex, thalamus, and interpeduncular nucleus and a substantial amount of binding in the amygdala, septum, and brain stem motor nuclei and locus ceruleus.[5] Neuronal acetylcholine receptors are composed of α and β subunits. There is much diversity in nicotinic cholinergic receptors with α2- through α9-subunits and β2- through β4-subunits identified in brain tissues.[6] The predominant neuronal receptor is α4, β2, which accounts for more than 90% of high-affinity binding in the rat brain. The α7-containing receptors are most likely responsible for α-bungarotoxin and low-affinity nicotine binding.[7] Different nicotinic cholinergic receptors are found in different areas of the brain and have different chemical conductances for sodium and calcium, different sensitivities to different nicotinic agonists, and result in correspondingly different pharmacological actions.[6] The diversity of nicotinic cholinergic receptors may explain the multiple effects of nicotine in humans and may present targets for specific nicotinic agonist or antagonist therapies.

When nicotine binds to nicotine receptors, allosteric changes occur such that there are several different functional states. These include the resting state, an activated state (channel open), and two desensitized states (channel closed).[8] The transition and persistence of receptors in the desensitized state is believed to explain tachyphylaxis and perhaps the observation that tolerance to nicotine is associated with an increased number of nicotinic cholinergic receptors (i.e., similar to a response to an antagonist in other receptor systems).[9] An increased number of nicotine receptors have been observed both in the brains of experimental animals during nicotine treatment and in the brains of human smokers at autopsy.[10]

Nicotinic receptors appear to be located both on cell bodies and at nerve termi-
nals. All nicotine receptors are permeable to calcium ions. Nicotinic receptor activation works, at least in part, and possibly in total, by facilitating the release of
neurotransmitters, including acetylcholine, norepinephrine, dopamine, serotonin,
β-endorphin, and glutamate. Nicotine also releases growth hormones, prolactin,
and adrenocorticotropic hormone (ACTH). Behavioral rewards from nicotine,
and perhaps nicotine addiction as well, appear to be linked to dopamine release,
particularly in the nigrostriatal region.[11] Most of the behavioral effects of nicotine
in people are believed to be mediated by actions on central nervous system receptors. However, activation of the brain by afferent receptors may also contribute.
Activation of nicotinic cholinergic receptors in the adrenal medulla release epinephrine, as well as β-endorphin.

Absorption of nicotine from tobacco and nicotine medications

Nicotine is distilled from burning tobacco and is carried proximally on tar
droplets (0.1–1.0 μM in diameter) that are inhaled and deposited in the small airways and alveoli. The absorption of nicotine across biological membranes depends on pH. The pH of smoke from flue-cured tobaccos found in most cigarettes
is acidic (pH 5.5). At this pH, the nicotine is primarily ionized. In this state, it
does not cross membranes rapidly. Consequently, there is little buccal absorption
of nicotine from cigarette smoke, even when it is held in the mouth.[12] The pH of
smoke from air-cured tobaccos, such as those in pipes, cigars, and a few European cigarettes, is alkaline (pH 8.5), and nicotine is primarily un-ionized. Smoke
from such products is well absorbed through the mouth.

When tobacco smoke reaches the small airways and alveoli of the lung, the
nicotine is absorbed rapidly, regardless of the pH of the smoke. Blood concentrations of nicotine rise quickly during cigarette smoking and peak at its completion
(Fig. 1-2). Presumably, the rapid absorption of nicotine from cigarette smoke
through the lung is the result of the huge surface area of the alveoli and small airways and the dissolution of nicotine into fluid of physiological pH, which facilitates transfer across cell membranes.

Chewing tobacco, snuff, and nicotine gum are buffered to an alkaline pH to facilitate the absorption of nicotine through the mucous membranes. Concentrations of nicotine in the blood rise gradually with use of smokeless tobacco and
tend to reach a plateau after about 30 minutes, with the levels persisting and de-
clining slowly over 2 hours or more (Fig. 1-2).

The process of cigarette smoking is complex, and the smoker can manipulate
the dose of nicotine on a puff-by-puff basis. Thus, the intake of nicotine from a
given product depends on the puff volume, the depth of inhalation, the extent of
dilution with room air, the rate of puffing, and intensity of puffing.[13] For certain

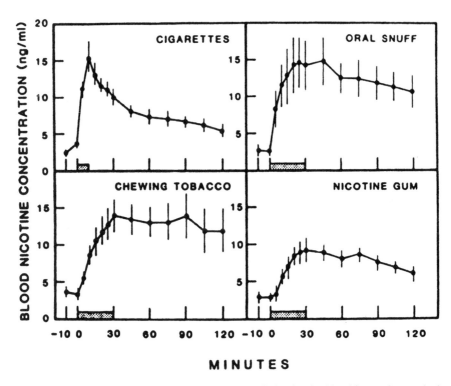

Figure 1-2. Mean (± SEM) blood concentrations of nicotine in 10 subjects who smoked cigarettes for 9 minutes (1 ⅓ cigarettes), used oral snuff (2.5 g), used chewing tobacco (mean, 7.9 g), and chewed nicotine gum (two 2-mg pieces). Shaded bars above the time axis indicate the period of exposure to tobacco or nicotine gum. (Reprinted from Benowitz et al.,[18] with permission of the publisher.)

"low tar" cigarettes, intake depends on whether ventilation holes in the filter are occluded by the smoker.[14]

Because of the complexity of the smoking process and use of smokeless tobacco products, the dose of nicotine taken in by the tobacco user cannot be predicted from the nicotine content of the tobacco or its absorption characteristics. To determine the dose, one needs to measure blood levels and know how fast the smoker eliminates nicotine. One study of 22 cigarette smokers, who smoked an average of 36 cigarettes per day (range, 20–62) found an average daily intake of 37 mg, with a wide range of 10–79 mg of nicotine.[15] The intake of nicotine per cigarette averaged 1.0 mg, but ranged from 0.37 to 1.56 mg. Similar results have been reported in other studies.[16,17] A study of nicotine intake from smokeless tobacco reported an average of 3.6 mg nicotine from 2.5 g of oral snuff and 4.6 mg nicotine from an average of 7.9 g of chewing tobacco when both were kept in the mouth for 30 minutes.[18]

Pharmacokinetics and metabolism of nicotine

Smoking is a unique form of systemic drug administration in that nicotine enters the circulation through the pulmonary rather than the portal or systemic venous circulations. It takes 10–19 seconds for nicotine to pass through the brain.[19] The lag time between smoking and the entry of nicotine into the brain is shorter than that observed when nicotine is injected intravenously. Nicotine enters the brain quickly, but brain levels decline rapidly thereafter as the drug is distributed to other body tissues.

Nicotine levels then fall due to uptake by peripheral tissues, then later due to elimination from the body. Arteriovenous differences during cigarette smoking are substantial, with arterial levels exceeding venous levels 6–10-fold.[20] The pharmacological relevance of this observation is that rapid delivery of nicotine results in a more intense pharmacological response, owing both to higher arterial levels entering the brain and to effects occurring rapidly, before there is adequate time for the development of tolerance.[21] Nicotine levels in the brain decline between cigarettes, providing an opportunity for resensitization of receptors so that positive reinforcement can, to some extent, occur with successive cigarettes despite the development of tolerance.

Nicotine crosses the placenta freely and has been found in amniotic fluid and in the umbilical cord blood of neonates.[22] It is found in breast milk and in the breast fluid of nonlactating women.[23,24] Its concentration in breast milk is so low that the dose of nicotine consumed by an infant is small and unlikely of physiological consequence.

Nicotine is rapidly and extensively metabolized, primarily in the liver, but also, to a small extent, in the lung. The level of renal excretion depends on urinary pH and urine flow and accounts for 2%–35% of the total elimination.[25] The metabolism of nicotine is described in more detail in Chapter 2 of this volume.

The half-life of nicotine averages 2 hours, although there is considerable individual variability (range, 1–4 hours).[26] Consistent with a 2-hour half-life, nicotine levels in the body rise during the first 6–8 hours and then plateau for the remainder of the day during regular smoking (Fig. 1-3). Nicotine levels fall overnight, but are still present at biologically significant levels when the smoker awakens after not smoking all night. Nicotine's primary metabolites are cotinine and nicotine-*N*-oxide (Fig. 1-1). Cotinine, because of its long half-life (16–20 hours),[27] is commonly used in surveys and treatment studies as a marker of nicotine intake.

Nicotine addiction

Most people who smoke cigarettes would like to quit.[28] Many of these people, who make up a group familiar to health care providers, either have a tobacco-

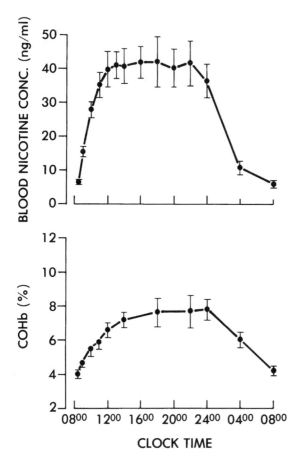

Figure 1-3. Mean (± SEM) blood nicotine and carboxyhemoglobin (COHb) concentrations in cigarette smokers. Subjects smoked cigarettes every half hour from 8:30 a.m. to 11:00 p.m., for a total of 30 cigarettes per day. (Adapted from Benowitz NL, Kuyt F,, & Jacob P III: Circadian blood nicotine concentrations during cigarette smoking. *Clinical Pharmacology and Therapeutics* 1982, 32: 758–764. with the permission of the publisher.)

related illness or recognize the threat posed by such illnesses but still cannot stop smoking. Their behavior is described well by a recent World Health Organization definition of drug dependence as "a behavioral pattern in which the use of a given psychoactive drug is given a sharply higher priority over other behaviors which once had a significantly higher value."[29] In other words, the drug has come to control behavior to an extent that is considered detrimental to the individual or society. Human use of nicotine from tobacco meets the criteria for drug dependence as presented by the U.S. Surgeon general (Table 1-1)

Recent studies in animals and humans have enhanced our understanding of

Table 1-1. Criteria for drug dependence

Primary Criteria
  Highly controlled or compulsive use
  Psychoactive effects
  Drug-reinforced behavior
Additional Criteria
  Addictive behavior often involves
    Stereotypical patterns of use
    Use despite harmful effects
    Relapse following abstinence
    Recurrent drug cravings
  Dependence-producing drugs often produce
    Tolerance
    Physical dependence
    Pleasant (euphoriant) effects

---

*From the 1987 Surgeon General's Report.[1]

nicotine addiction. Animals, including rats and squirrel monkeys, and humans will self-administer intravenous nicotine. Intravenous nicotine is self-administered in these studies at dose levels comparable with those taken in when people smoke cigarettes. Self-administration occurs for other addicting drugs and provides a method for exploring mechanisms of reinforcement. Studies in the rat suggest that the mesolimbic dopamine system is central to the reinforcing effects of nicotine.[11] The mesolimbic system projects from the ventral tegmental area of the midbrain to the nucleus accumbens and is known to be involved in reinforcement for other drugs of abuse such as cocaine. High-affinity binding of labeled nicotine to cell bodies and terminal fields of the mesolimbic neurons and expression of mRNAs for α-3, α-4, α5-, and β2-subunits in mesolimbic neurons has been demonstrated.[30] Nicotine increases firing of ventral tegmental area neurons and facilitates release of neurotransmitters in this system. Supporting the role of dopaminergic neurons in sustaining self-administration are studies with dopamine antagonists and chemical lesions of the dopaminergic system using 6-hydroxydopamine, both of which abolish self-administration.[31] In addition, nicotine antagonists, such as chlorosondamine, infused directly into the ventral segmental area or the nucleus accumbens reduce self-administration.

Humans have been shown to like and self-administer intravenous nicotine, and the reinforcing effects and the self-administration can be blocked by pretreatment with the nicotine antagonist mecamylamine.[32] In smokers, nicotine self-administration appears to be motivated by both positive reinforcement and negative reinforcement. Positive reinforcing effects that are reported include relaxation, reduced stress, enhanced vigilance, improved cognitive function, mood modulation, and lower body weight. Negative reinforcement refers to the relief of nicotine withdrawal symptoms in the context of physical dependence. Withdrawal symptoms are well documented to include nervousness, restlessness, irritability, anxiety, impaired concentration, impaired cognitive function, increased appetite, and weight gain.[33] It is difficult to separate reported positive reinforcement from relief of withdrawal symptoms in smokers. Recent studies of nonsmokers, however, indicate some enhancement of cognitive function and less of a decrement in performance with repetitive tasks after nicotine.[34] Of note is that performance of smokers (compared with deprived smokers) in a complex behavioral task has also been reported to be impaired by nicotine.[35] Some smokers report that smoking helps relieve depression and other affective disorders, and, conversely, some smokers become severely depressed after stopping smoking.[36] Neurochemical effects of nicotine, including release of dopamine, norepinephrine, and serotonin, resemble effects of some antidepressant medications. Conceivably, nicotine is self-administered by some smokers to treat affective disorders. In addition to nicotine-related effects, there is evidence that sensory stimulation induced by nicotine contributes to the satisfaction from smoking.[37] This, however, may be a short-term conditioned response and is not likely to maintain nicotine self-administration in the long term.

In smokers, nicotine produces electroencephalographic activation including increased beta power, decreased alpha and theta power, and increased alpha frequency.[38] Changes in the opposite direction are seen during tobacco abstinence, and these changes are rapidly reversed by nicotine in any form. Nicotine has been shown to increase regional cerebral glucose metabolism in areas that are also shown to have high-affinity nicotine binding, possibly representing a neuroanatomical correlate of nicotine effects.[39]

Addiction to nicotine depends on the rate and route of nicotine dosing. Inhalation of nicotine via cigarette smoking appears to be the most addictive method of dosing. After inhalation, nicotine passes rapidly into the arterial blood stream and then into the brain, resulting in a transient exposure of the brain to high levels of nicotine. This exposure results in relatively intense central nervous system effects that occur in close temporal proximity to smoking, an ideal situation for behavioral reinforcement. As discussed, arterial levels of nicotine are severalfold higher than venous levels after smoking, and arterial levels far exceed those that would be tolerated with nicotine dosing via a systemic route. Transiently high nicotine levels in the brain, which subsequently fall between cigarettes, allow time for resensitization of brain nicotinic receptors. Thus, nicotine from sequential cigarettes is capable of overcoming tolerance to produce further pharmacological effects. Finally, rapid delivery of nicotine to the brain allows the smoker to titrate the dose of nicotine from a cigarette to achieve a particular desired effect without toxicity.

Endocrine and metabolic effects of nicotine

Nicotine has important cardiovascular, endocrine, and metabolic effects. The cardiovascular effects of nicotine are described in detail in other chapters in this volume.

Metabolic effects of nicotine are of interest in regard to effects on body weight and serum lipids, which could affect cardiovascular disease risk. On average, cigarette smokers weigh 4 kg less than nonsmokers, and, when smokers quit, their body weight increases, on average, that amount.[40] Lower body weight seems to be maintained primarily by an increased metabolic rate, with concomitant appetite suppression, evidenced by the absence of a compensatory increase in caloric intake that would be expected when metabolic rate increases.[41] Both cigarette smoking and intravenous nicotine dosing have been shown to increase the metabolic rate.[42] Smoking cessation is associated with an increase in appetite and caloric intake, particularly of sweet foods, resulting in an increase in body weight over 6–12 months.[41] Subsequently, caloric intake is reduced and returns to baseline, indicating a new set point for body weight. The mechanism for the nicotine-mediated increase in metabolic rate has not been fully elucidated. Catecholamine release is most likely involved, as the increase in metabolic rate is inhibited by β-blockers.[43]

Nicotine, via release of catecholamines, induces lipolysis and releases free fatty acids into the plasma. Cigarette smoking in humans and nicotine administration in animals has been shown to substantially enhance free fatty acid turnover.[44] Fatty acids are primarily taken up by the liver, which might be expected to increase the synthesis of very-low-density lipoproteins. Increased low-density lipoproteins and very-low-density lipoproteins and decreased high-density lipoprotein levels have been reported in smokers.[45] It is conceivable that the effects of nicotine could contribute to the lipid abnormalities of cigarette smoking. Such abnormalities have not, however, been seen in individuals using nicotine replacement therapies.[46]

Nicotine has a variety of endocrine effects that are of biological interest. The release of neurotransmitters that could influence the psychotropic effects and addiction to nicotine have been discussed previously. Cigarette smoking, presumably via the effects of nicotine, has been shown to increase ACTH and cortisol release.[47,48] Excessive cortisol release could have effects on mood and could contribute to osteoporosis.

Nicotine can release β-endorphins.[48] It has antinociceptive effects in animals and possibly in humans, effects that could be mediated, at least in part, by endorphin release,[49,50] although there is also evidence for antinociception via spinal and brain stem neural pathways. Release of catecholamines and endorphins may also contribute to the effects of nicotine to reduce the fluid extravasation response to bradykinin from the synovium in the joints of rats.[51] Inhibition of synovial fluid extravasation suggests that nicotine might contribute to inflammatory arthritis.

Cigarette smoking is a risk factor for osteoporosis.[52] The mechanism is not clear but is likely to involve the lower body weight of smokers (which is mediated by nicotine) and possibly by the antiestrogenic effects of cigarette smoking.[53] Recent studies have indicated that estrogen and steroid levels in smokers are normal, although estrogen levels in postmenopausal women on estrogen replacement therapy who smoke cigarettes are lower than those of nonsmokers,[54,55] and smoking eliminates the protective effect of oral estrogens for hip fracture. The latter may be an effect of cigarette smoking and resulting enzyme induction on estrogen metabolism rather than an effect of nicotine. However, animal studies indicate that nicotine can reduce bone mass, although the mechanism has not been determined.[56] Corticosteroids reduce the sensitivity to nicotine in mice, at least in part by reducing nicotinic binding, and nicotine-mediated corticosteroid release is suspected to contribute to nicotine tolerance.[57]

Conclusions

Nicotine maintains tobacco addiction and has the therapeutic utility to aid in smoking cessation and to treat other medical diseases. Nicotine acts on nicotinic cholinergic receptors, which demonstrate diversity in subunit structure, function, and distribution within the nervous system, mediating the complex actions of nicotine described in tobacco smokers. Nicotine affects most organ systems in the body. The nature and intensity of effects of nicotine are influenced by the rate and route of dosing and by the development of tolerance. Effects of nicotine are most intense, and addiction is most likely to occur, with rapid dosing, as occurs with cigarette smoking. Addiction to nicotine occurs as a consequence of both positive reinforcement and seeking to relieve withdrawal symptoms that occur in the context of physical dependence. The most important toxicity of nicotine is the maintenance of addiction to tobacco use, which results in many millions of premature deaths and other severe illnesses yearly. Whether nicotine has direct toxicity independent of causing addiction is the subject of the remainder of this volume.

Acknowledgments

I thank Kaye Welch for editorial assistance. Preparation of this chapter was supported in part by National Institute on Drug Abuse, National Institutes of Health grants DA02277 and DA01696.

References

1. Department of Health and Human Services, P. H. S: *The Health Consequences of Smoking: Nicotine Addiction.* A Report of the Surgeon General. DHHS (CDC) Publication No. 88-8406. Washington, DC: Government Printing Office, 1988.

2. Benowitz NL: Cigarette smoking and nicotine addiction. *Medical Clinics of North America* 1992, 76:415–437.

3. Benowitz NL: Pharmacology of nicotine: Addiction and therapeutics. *Annual Review of Pharmacology Toxicology* 1996, 36:597–613.

4. Changeux JP, Galzi JL, Devillers-Thiery A, Betrand D: The functional architecture of the acetylcholine nicotinic receptor explored by affinity labeling and site-directed mutatgenesis. *Quarterly Reviews of Biophysics* 1992, 25:395–432.

5. Clarke PBS, Schwartz RD, Paul SM, Pert CB, Pert, A: Nicotinic binding in rat brain: Autoradiographic comparison of [^{3}H]acetylcholine, [^{3}H]nicotine and [^{125}I]α-bungarotoxin. *Journal of Neuroscience* 1985, 5:1307–1315.

6. McGehee DS, Role LW: Physiological diversity of nicotinic acetylcholine receptors expressed by vertebrate neurons. *Annual Reviews of Physiology* 1995, 57:521–546.

7. Seguela P, Wadiche J, Dineley-Miller K, Dani JA, Patrick JW: Molecular cloning, functional properties, and distribution of rat brain α7: A nicotinic cation channel highly permeable to calcium. *Journal of Neuroscience* 1993, 13:596–604.

8. Lena C, Changeux J-P: Allosteric modulations of the nicotinic acetylcholine receptor. *Trends in Neuroscience* 1993, 16:181–186.

9. Wonnacott S: The paradox of nicotinic acetylcholine receptor upregulation by nicotine. TIPS 1990, 11:216–219.

10. Benwell MEM, Balfour DJK, Anderson JM: Evidence that tobacco smoking increases the density of (-)-[^{3}H]nicotine binding sites in human brain. *Journal of Neurochemistry* 1988, 50:1243–1247.

11. Corrigall WA, Coen KM, Adamson KL: Self-administered nicotine activates the mesolimbic dopamine system through the ventral tegmental area. *Brain Research* 1994, 653:278–284.

12. Gori GB, Benowitz NL, Lynch CJ: Mouth versus deep airways absorption of nicotine in cigarette smokers. *Pharmacology Biochemistry, and Behavior* 1986, 25: 1181–1184.

13. Herning RI, Jones RT, Benowitz NL, Mines AH: How a cigarette is smoked determines nicotine blood levels. *Clinical Pharmacology and Therapeutics* 1983, 33: 84–90.

14. Zacny JP, Stitzer ML, Yingling JE: Cigarette filter vent blocking: Effects on smoking topography and carbon monoxide exposure. *Pharmacology, Biochemistry, and Behavior* 1986, 25:1245–1452.

15. Benowitz NL, Jacob P III: Daily intake of nicotine during cigarette smoking. *Clinical Pharmacology and Therapeutics* 1984, 35:499–504.

16. Armitage AK, Dollery CT, George CF, Houseman TH, Lewis PJ, Turner DM: Absorption and metabolism of nicotine from cigarettes. *British Medical Journal* 1975, 4: 313–316.

17. Feyerabend C, Ings RMJ, Russell MAH: Nicotine pharmacokinetics and its application to intake from smoking. *British Journal of Clinical Pharmacology* 1985, 19: 239–247.

18. Benowitz NL, Porchet H, Sheiner L, Jacob P III: Nicotine absorption and cardiovas-

cular effects with smokeless tobacco use: Comparison with cigarettes and nicotine gum. *Clinical Pharmacology and Therapeutics* 1988, 44:23–28.

19. Benowitz NL: Clinical pharmacology of inhaled drugs of abuse: Implications in understanding nicotine dependence. In Chiang CN, Hawks RL (eds): *Research Findings on Smoking of Abused Substances.* NIDA Research Monograph 99. Washington, DC: Supterintendent of Documents, 1990, pp 12–29.

20. Henningfield JE, Stapleton JM, Benowitz NL, Grayson RF, London ED: Higher levels of nicotine in arterial than in venous blood after cigarette smoking. *Drug Alcohol Dependence* 1993, 33:23–29.

21. Porchet HC, Benowitz NL, Sheiner LB, Copeland JR: Apparent tolerance to the acute effect of nicotine results in part from distribution kinetics. *Journal of Clinical Investigation* 1987, 80:1466–1471.

22. Luck W, Nau H: Exposure of the fetus, neonate, and nursed infant to nicotine and cotinine from maternal smoking. *New England Journal of Medicine* 1984, 311:672.

23. Petrakis NL, Gruenke LD, Beelen TC, Castagnoli N, Craig JC: Nicotine in breast fluid of nonlactating women. *Science* 1978, 199:303–305.

24. Luck W, Nau H: Nicotine and cotinine concentrations in the milk of smoking mothers: Influence of cigarette consumption and diurnal variation. *European Journal of Pediatrics* 1987, 146:21–26.

25. Benowitz NL, Jacob P III: Nicotine renal excretion rate influences nicotine intake during cigarette smoking. *Journal of Pharmacology and Experimental Therapeutics* 1985, 234:153–155.

26. Benowitz NL, Jacob P III, Jones RT, Rosenberg J: Interindividual variability in the metabolism and cardiovascular effects of nicotine in man. *Journal of Pharmacology and Experimental Theraputics* 1982, 221:368–372.

27. Benowitz NL, Kuyt F, Jacob P III, Jones RT, Osman AL: Cotinine disposition and effects. *Clinical Pharmacology and Therapeutics* 1983., 309:139–142.

28. Orleans CT: Understanding and promoting smoking cessation: Overview and guidelines for physician intervention. *Annual Review of Medicine* 1985, 36:51–61.

29. Edwards G, Arif A, Hodgson R: Nomenclature and classification of drug and alcohol-related problems: A shortened version of a WHO memorandum. *British Journal of Addiction* 1982, 77:3–20.

30. Clarke PBS, Pert A: Autoradiographic evidence for nicotine receptors on nigrostriatal and mesolimbic dopaminergic neurons. *Brain Research* 1985, 348:355–358.

31. Corrigall WA, Coen KM, Franklin KBJ, Clarke PBS: The mesolimbic dopamine system is implicated in the reinforcing effects of nicotine. *Psychopharmacology* 1992, 107:285–289.

32. Henningfield JE: Behavioral pharmacology of cigarette smoking. In Thompson T, Dews PB, Barrett JE (eds): *Advances in Behavioral Pharmacology* New York: Academic Press, 1984, pp 131–210.

33. Hughes JR, Hatsukami D: Signs and symptoms of tobacco withdrawal. *Archives of General Psychiatry* 1986, 43:289–294.

34. LeHouezec J, Halliday R, Benowitz NL, Callaway E, Naylor H, Herzig K: A low dose of subcutaneous nicotine improves information processing in nonsmokers. *Psychopharmacology* 1994, 114:628–634.

35. Spilich GJ, June L, Renner J: Cigarette smoking and cognitive performance. *British Journal of Addiction* 1992, 87:1313–1326.

36. Covey LS, Glassman AH, Stetner F: Depression and depressive symptoms in smoking cessation. *Comprehensive Psychiatry* 1990, 31:350–354.

37. Rose JE, Behm FM, Levin ED: Role of nicotine dose and sensory cues in the regulation of smoke intake. *Pharmacology Biochemistry, and Behavior* 1993, 44:891–900.
38. Pickworth WB, Herning RI, Henningfield JE: Spontaneous EEG changes during tobacco abstinence and nicotine substitution in human volunteers. *Journal of Pharmacology and Experimental Therapeutics* 1989, 251:976–982.
39. McNamara D, Larson DM, Rapoport SI, Soncrant TT: Preferential metabolic activation of subcortical brain areas by acute administration of nicotine to rats. *Journal of Cerebral Blood Flow and Metabolism* 1990, 10:48–56.
40. Williamson DF, Madans J, Anda RF, Kleinman JC, Giovino GA, Byers T: Smoking cessation and severity of weight gain in a national cohort. *New England Journal of Medicine* 1991, 324:739–745.
41. Perkins KA: Metabolic effects of cigarette smoking. *Journal of Applied Physiology* 1992, 72:401–409.
42. Arcavi L, Jacob P III, Hellerstein M, Benowitz NL: Divergent tolerance to metabolic and cardiovascular effects of nicotine in smokers with low and high levels of cigarette consumption. *Clinical Pharmacology and Therapeutics* 1994, 56:55–64.
43. Wahren J: *Nicotine, cigarette smoking and energy expenditure in humans* (abstract). European Chemical Society Conference on Nicotine, Visby, Sweden, 1990.
44. Hellerstein MK, Benowitz NL, Neese RA, Schwartz J, Hoh R, Jacob P III, Hsieh J, Faix D: Effects of cigarette smoking and its cessation on lipid metabolism and energy expenditure in heavy smokers. *Journal of Clinical of Investigation* 1994, 93: 265–272.
45. Craig WY, Palomaki GE, Haddow JE: Cigarette smoking and serum lipid and lipoprotein concentrations: An analysis of published data. *British Medical Journal* 1989, 298:784–788.
46. Quensel M, Agardh C-D, Nilsson-Ehle P: Nicotine does not affect plasma lipoprotein concentrations in healthy men. *Scandinavian Journal of Clinical and Laboratory Investigation* 1989, 49:149–153.
47. Baron JA, Comi RJ, Cryns V, Brinck-Johnsen T, Mercer NG: The effect of cigarette smoking on adrenal cortical hormones. *Journal of Pharmacology and Experimental Therapeutics* 1995, 272:151–155.
48. Seyler LE, Pomerleau OF, Fertig JB, Hunt D, Parker K: Pituitary hormone response to cigarette smoking. *Pharmacology Biochemistry, and Behavior* 1986, 24:159–162.
49. Pomerleau OF, Turk DC, Fertig JB: The effects of cigarette smoking on pain and anxiety. *Addictive Behaviors* 1984, 9:265–271.
50. Rogers DT, Iwamoto ET: Multiple spinal mediators in parenteral nicotine-induced antinociception. *Journal of Pharmacology and Experimental Therapeutics* 1993, 267:341–349.
51. Miao FJ, Dallman MF, Benowitz NL, Basbaum AI, Levine JD: Adrenal medullary modulation of the inhibition of bradykinin-induced plasma extravasation by intrathecal nicotine. *Journal of Pharmacology and Expeimental Therapeutics* 1993, 53:6–14.
52. Hopper JL, Seeman E: The bone density of female twins discordant for tobacco use. *New England Journal of Medicine* 1994, 330:387–392.
53. Baron JA, LeVecchia C, Levi F: The antiestrogenic effect of cigarette smoking in women. *American Journal of Obstetrics and Gynecology* 1990, 162:502–514.
54. Cassidenti DL, Pike MC, Vijod AG, Stanczyk FZ, Lobo RA: A reevaluation of estrogen status in postmenopausal women who smoke. *American Journal of Obstetrics and Gynecology* 1992, 166:1444–1448.
55. Kiel DP, Baron JA, Anderson JJ, Hannan MT, Felson DT: Smoking eliminates the pro-

tective effect of oral estrogens on the risk for hip fracture among women. *Annuls of Internal Medicine* 1992, 116:716–721.

56. Broulik PD, Jarab J: The effect of chronic nicotine administration on bone mineral content in mice. *Hormone and Metabolic Research* 1993, 25:219–221.

57. Pauly JR, Collins AC: An autoradiographic analysis of alterations in nicotinic cholinergic receptors following 1 week of corticosterone supplementation. *Neuroendocrinology* 1993, 57:262–271.

Part **I**

Nicotine
and Cardiovascular Disease

Cigarette smoking is a major cause of cardiovascular disease. It accelerates atherogenesis, which results in cerebrovascular disease, aortic aneurysm, and peripheral occlusive vascular disease at a considerably younger age in smokers than nonsmokers. Cigarette smoking also increases the risk of acute cardiovascular events, including sudden death, acute myocardial infarction, and stroke, and increases the risk of reocclusion of coronary or peripheral vessels after graft surgery or angioplasty.

Nicotine has effects on cardiovascular physiology. It increases blood pressure and force of contraction of the heart. In addition, nicotine affects metabolism, increasing free fatty acid levels. Nicotine poisoning, as has occurred after exposure to nicotine insecticides, can produce cardiovascular collapse and death. Not surprisingly, nicotine is suspected to contribute to smoking-related cardiovascular disease. Thus, there is concern that nicotine replacement therapy, especially with concomitant cigarette smoking, might cause or aggravate cardiovascular disease. In 1992, several individuals were reported to have suffered acute myocardial infarction while using nicotine patches and smoking. This cluster of cases was investigated by the Food and Drug Administration, which determined that nicotine patches were not the cause of death, but many physicians and scientists have had lingering concerns. The mechanisms by which nicotine could promote cardiovascular disease are reviewed and studies of the safety of nicotine administered to patients with cardiovascular disease are examined in Part I.

Chapter 2

Cardiovascular Toxicity of Nicotine: Pharmacokinetic and Pharmacodynamic Considerations

NEAL L. BENOWITZ

There is great interest in nicotine medications for smoking cessation and long-term maintenance of cessation. In addition, nicotine medications have been proposed as possible treatments for conditions such as depression, Alzheimer's disease, and Parkinson's disease. The investigation of nicotine as a discrete agent is vital to determining its potential benefits and clarifying associated risks.

The toxicity of nicotine must be considered in the context of what concentrations of nicotine are acting on body organs and over what time course the nicotine has been delivered. In determining the relevance of animal research to human exposure data, it is important to examine blood or organ concentrations of nicotine and rates, routes, and duration of dosing. It is also important to distinguish the toxicity of tobacco, which exposes an individual to thousands of potential toxins, from exposure to nicotine per se. This chapter summarizes pharmacokinetic and pharmacodynamic factors that should be considered in understanding the toxicity and safety of nicotine.

Mechanisms of cardiovascular toxicity of nicotine

Discerning the general mechanisms of concern with respect to nicotine cardiovascular toxicity is critical. One of the major effects of nicotine is activation of the sympathetic nervous system, which is a useful marker of nicotine's effects on the cardiovascular system.

Cigarette smoking is well known to be associated with accelerated atherosclerosis and increased incidence of cardiovascular disease, including acute myocardial infarction, sudden death, stroke, aortic aneurysms, and peripheral vascular disease.[1] Many toxins are believed to contribute to smoking-related cardiovascular disease, including carbon monoxide, oxidant gases, and nicotine. Some, but not all, characteristics of tobacco-related disease seem to be nicotine related.

Nicotine increases central nervous system sympathetic outflow, adrenal release of catecholamines, and local release of catecholamines from vascular nerve endings.[2] The net result is heart rate acceleration, increased myocardial contractility, constriction of some blood vessels, including coronary arteries and cutaneous blood vessels, and a small increase in blood pressure (Fig. 2-1).

Nicotine could precipitate or aggravate acute coronary ischemic events by increasing myocardial work, and therefore nutrient demand, while reducing nutrient supply through coronary vasoconstriction. Catecholamine release may also precipitate or aggravate ischemia-induced arrhythmias, leading to sudden arrhythmic death. Other possible adverse cardiovascular effects of nicotine include injury to endothelial cells, induction of an atherogenic lipid profile, and promotion of thrombosis. These effects are discussed later in this chapter, as well as by other authors in this volume.

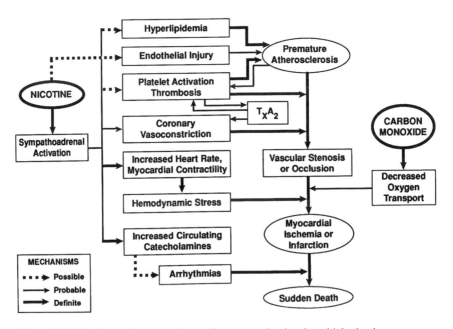

Figure 2-1. Nicotine and coronary heart disease: mechanism by which nicotine may cause or aggravate cardiovascular disease. (Reprinted from Benowitz,[17] with permission of the publisher.)

Implications of rate of nicotine dosing

Rapid dosing of nicotine, as in cigarette smoking, produces more intense cardio-vascular effects than does more gradual dosing, as with nicotine gum or transder-mal nicotine.[3] This is because arterial nicotine levels are much higher after rapid dosing, and with a rapid rise in levels there is less time for the development of acute tolerance.

After smoking a cigarette, nicotine is absorbed rapidly from the lungs into the pulmonary venous circulation and then into the heart, from which it is pumped in the arterial circulation to various body organs. Arterial blood nicotine concentra-tions after cigarette smoking may be as high as 100 ng/ml (6×10^{-7} M).[4] Since organs such as the heart and brain may have partition coefficients of 2 or 3, con-centrations of nicotine in these organs may be as high as 200–300 ng/ml after a cigarette.[5] Venous blood nicotine concentrations are typically 20%–30% of those of arterial concentrations. Venous levels reflect the balance of efflux of nicotine from body tissues and elimination by the liver and kidneys.

Most published research has concentrated on venous nicotine levels, which substantially underestimate the nicotine levels in body organs, and thus at nico-tine receptors, after cigarette smoking. As a general principle, the faster a drug is absorbed, the greater will be the difference between arterial and venous con-centrations. Therefore, in contrast to smoking a cigarette, the gradual absorp-tion of nicotine from transdermal nicotine patches should result in very similar arterial and venous concentrations, so typical organ exposures would be in the range of 20–30 ng/ml. Nicotine nasal spray, which is absorbed faster than nico-tine gum or nicotine patches, but more slowly than nicotine from cigarette smoking, produces an intermediate degree of arteriovenous difference in nico-tine concentration.

Heart rate acceleration has been used as a continuous measure of nicotine-me-diated sympathetic nervous system stimulation. Using heart rate as a marker, it has been shown that rapid dosing produces a much greater effect than does slower administration of a similar dose of nicotine.[3] Likewise, the subjective effects of smoking a cigarette are greater than the subjective effects after nicotine exposure from chewing nicotine gum, which is, in turn, greater than that after transdermal nicotine patch application.[6] Abuse liability appears greater with nicotine delivery systems than with nicotine delivered more rapidly.

Nicotine induces substantial but not complete tolerance to cardiovascular effects

Tolerance to the noxious effects of nicotine is well known. The novice smoker of-ten becomes nauseated after the first few cigarettes, but soon develops complete tolerance to such effects. Likewise, substantial tolerance develops to some of the cardiovascular effects of nicotine.[7] Mechanisms of tolerance development include receptor desensitization and, for cardiovascular effects, probably some homeostatic compensation. Conditioned tolerance to cardiovascular effects of nicotine has also been described in humans.[8]

Acute tolerance to the heart rate accelerating effect of nicotine has been studied by examining the relationship between venous blood nicotine concentrations and heart rate acceleration over the course of an intravenous infusion.[9] While plasma nicotine concentrations rise steadily over 30 minutes during the infusion, heart rate acceleration peaks at 5 minutes, and then plateaus. As plasma nicotine concentrations fall, the extent of heart rate acceleration at any given plasma nicotine concentration is less than the extent of heart rate acceleration in the rising phase, consistent with the development of acute tolerance.

However, the development of tolerance to heart rate acceleration is not complete. During daily cigarette smoking or prolonged intravenous infusion of nicotine, heart rate remains persistently above baseline.[10,11] It is estimated by pharmacodynamic modeling that the extent of heart rate acceleration at steady state is 20% of that which would have occurred at a given blood nicotine concentration in the absence of tolerance.[7] Thus, no matter how long a person is exposed to nicotine, there is persistent sympathetic nervous system activation. This may be an important factor in the causation of vascular injury.

Nicotine dose–response relationships

The development of substantial but partial tolerance has implications for understanding the nicotine dose–response relationship. Both theoretical prediction and experimental studies describe robust nicotine effects at relatively low exposure levels, but then relatively small increments in response as the dose or concentration increases.[7,10,11] Thus, higher doses of nicotine produce little, if any, greater heart rate acceleration than do lower doses.

Two experimental studies illustrate this point. In one study, heart rate was measured over 24 hours while smokers were smoking 30 cigarettes per day of either a high nicotine content or a low nicotine content cigarette.[10] The differences in plasma nicotine concentrations achieved were fourfold, but the time course and degree of heart rate acceleration was similar in both smoking conditions. Heart rate increased after the first few cigarettes of the day and then remained elevated (compared with a tobacco abstinence condition) for 24 hours. The average increase in heart rate was seven beats per minute over the day.

A second study examined the effects of intravenous nicotine on the intake of nicotine from cigarette smoking.[11] In the combined intravenous and smoking condition, plasma nicotine concentrations were about 175% of those seen in the smoking alone condition. Despite these high levels, there was no greater heart rate acceleration or urinary catecholamine release in the combined intravenous and smoking condition than in smoking alone condition or intravenous nicotine alone condition. Both of these studies demonstrate the flat dose–response relationship for nicotine, which has implications for understanding the toxicity of nicotine at different dose levels and for the toxicity of simultaneous nicotine administration and cigarette smoking.

Nicotine metabolites

Nicotine is extensively metabolized, primarily in the liver (Fig. 2-2, 2-3). The proximate metabolite is cotinine, which accounts for, on average, 80%–90% of nicotine metabolism.[12] A minor metabolite is nicotine-N-oxide, accounting for about 5% of nicotine metabolism. Cotinine is, in turn, metabolized to *trans*-3'-hydroxycotinine, the latter of which is the most abundant nicotine metabolite in the urine. Nicotine, cotinine, and *trans*-3'-hydroxycotinine form to glucuronide conjugates, which are excreted in the urine.

With regular nicotine exposure, plasma levels of cotinine average about 15 times those of nicotine. Plasma levels of trans-3'-hydroxycotinine are about three times higher than those of nicotine.[13] Little is known of the long-term cardiovas-

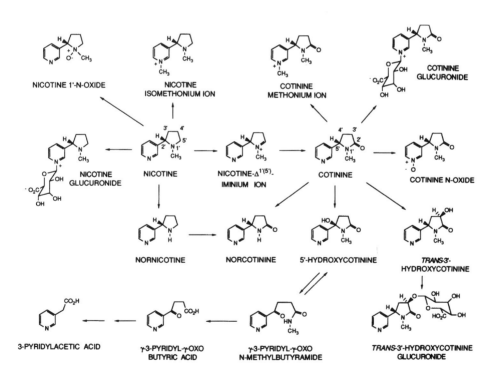

Figure 2-2. Nicotine metabolic pathways and structures. (Reprinted with permission from Benowitz et al.,[12] with permission of the publisher.)

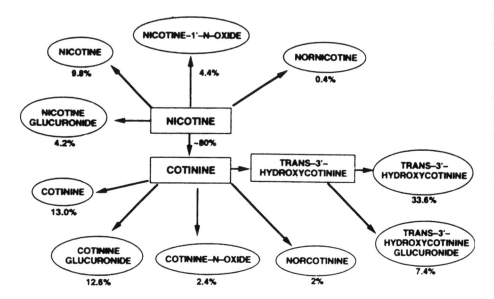

Figure 2-3. Quantitative scheme of nicotine metabolism. (Reprinted from Benowitz et al.[12] with permission of the publisher.)

cular effects of cotinine or *trans*-3'-hydroxycotinine. While there appears to be little acute effect of cotinine on heart rate and blood pressure, cotinine has been shown in vitro to inhibit the metabolism of some steroids, including aldosterone.[14,15] In any case, when considering the chronic effects of nicotine and nicotine toxicity, the pharmacology of nicotine metabolites needs to be considered as well.

Nicotine and thrombosis

A particular concern regarding nicotine and cardiovascular disease is the question of enhanced thrombosis. Smoking induces a hypercoagulable state, and acute thrombosis is an important factor in causing acute myocardial infarction and stroke. Platelet activation is likely also to contribute to accelerated atherogenesis. A brief summary of one study of nicotine and thrombosis is addressed in the following text.

This study was a crossover study of smokers studied in 5–day blocks, during which the subjects smoked cigarettes (20 per day), wore transdermal nicotine systems delivering 21 mg over 24 hours or wore placebo patches.[16] The sequence of treatment conditions was balanced. Platelet activation was assessed by measuring the release of platelet granule components, platelet factor IV, and β-thromboglobulin, and by measuring metabolites of thromboxane A_2, a prostaglandin released by platelets when they are activated.

Despite similar daily exposure to nicotine, the smoking condition produced significantly greater increases in thromboxane A_2 metabolite excretion, β-thromboglobulin and platelet factor IV, and catecholamines than the nicotine patch condition. The nicotine and placebo patch conditions had similar values. Thus, this study suggests that nicotine, at least absorbed transdermally, does not activate platelets, whereas cigarette smoking does. At this time, the possibility that rapid delivery of nicotine is responsible for platelet activation cannot be excluded. However, it is more likely that other substances in tobacco smoke, such as glycoproteins or oxidant gases, are responsible for the hypercoagulable state of smokers. This observation reinforces the idea that the effects of cigarette smoking are not necessarily effects of nicotine and that the safety profile of nicotine is likely to be much different than that of cigarette smoking.

Conclusions

Adverse effects of nicotine on the cardiovascular system and perhaps other organ systems are believed to result primarily from activation of the sympathetic nervous system. The hemodynamic consequences of sympathetic nervous system activation include increased heart rate and blood pressure, thereby resulting in greater myocardial work and oxygen requirement and in coronary vasoconstriction, which reduces myocardial oxygen supply. Nicotine has also been purported to activate platelets and to adversely affect blood lipids, which could both promote atherosclerosis and increase the risk of acute coronary events.

The intensity of nicotine effect depends on the rate of delivery of nicotine via the systemic circulation. This is because more rapid delivery results in higher arterial concentrations of nicotine as well as more rapid presentation to target organs, allowing less time for development of acute tolerance. Thus, the intensity of effects is likely to be greatest for nicotine delivered via cigarette smoking, intermediate for nicotine nasal spray, and lowest for nicotine gum and transdermal nicotine. The maximal blood concentration of nicotine in arterial blood after cigarette smoking is about 100 ng/ml (6×10^{-7} M). This level needs to be considered when extrapolating pharmacological studies from animals to humans.

Tolerance develops to sympathomimetic effects of nicotine, such as heart rate acceleration. Tolerance develops rapidly, but is not complete. At a steady-state level of 25 ng/ml nicotine, heart rate acceleration remains above baseline at about 20% of the level that would have been expected had tolerance not developed. This may be seen as a persistent increase in heart rate of about seven beats per minute during regular tobacco use compared with no nicotine exposure. The dose–response relationship for nicotine cardiovascular effects is relatively flat. Thus, even low doses could theoretically have adverse effects. Conversely, higher doses are not necessarily more toxic than lower doses.

A major mechanism of acute cardiovascular events is thrombosis, which is enhanced by cigarette smoking. The role of nicotine in promoting thrombosis has not yet been determined. Transdermal nicotine and snuff use, both of which deliver nicotine to the circulation slowly, do not appear to activate platelets, whereas cigarette smoking does. Thus, nicotine per se does not explain platelet activation. Whether nicotine delivered rapidly will activate platelets remains to be determined.

Given the current data covering tobacco and cardiovascular toxicity, questions still arise about which specific components of tobacco-related disease are related to nicotine. With the availability of over-the-counter nicotine replacement products, follow-up studies may be able to ascertain, in human subjects, a more exact causal relationship between nicotine and tobacco-related diseases.

It is unclear whether recommending the patch versus recommending abstinence is the preferred course of action for those trying to quit smoking. The answer would be, most likely, different depending on the health status of those facing this decision. For instance, those attempting smoking cessation who have had acute myocardial infarction or unstable angina, or women who are pregnant, raise questions about the possible injurious impact of nicotine administered in a replacement medication versus the benefit of abstinence (and the lower likelihood of sustained quitting had no nicotine replacement been administered). In addition, variables such as dosage and acute versus chronic treatment need to be considered because what may not be harmful over the course of a 6-month period may be harmful over a 20-year period. The same considerations would have to be dealt with if it were determined that nicotine could be used as an agent to improve the health status of those with, for instance, depression.

Acknowledgments

Research was supported in part by grants DA02277 and DA01696 from the National Institute on Drug Abuse, National Institutes of Health. The editorial assistance of Kaye Welch is greatly appreciated.

References

1. McBride PE: The health consequences of smoking: cardiovascular diseases. *Medical Clinics of North America* 1992, 76:333–353.
2. Benowitz NL: Pharmacologic aspects of cigarette smoking and nicotine addiction. *New England Journal of Medicine* 1988, 319:1318–1330.
3. Porchet HC, Benowitz NL, Sheiner LB, Copeland JR: Apparent tolerance to the acute effect of nicotine results in part from distribution kinetics. *Journal of Clinical Investigation* 1987, 80:1466–1471.
4. Henningfield JE, Stapleton JM, Benowitz NL, Grayson RF, London ED: Higher levels of nicotine in arterial than in venous blood after cigarette smoking. *Drug and Alcohol Dependence* 1993, 33:23–29.
5. Benowitz NL, Porchet H, Jacob P III: Pharmacokinetics, metabolism, and pharmacodynamics of nicotine. In Wonnacotts S, Russell MAH, Stolerman IP (eds): *Nicotine*

Psychopharmacology: Molecular, Cellular, and Behavioral Aspects. Oxford: Oxford University Press, 1990, pp 42–157.

6. Henningfield JE, Keenan RM: Nicotine delivery kinetics and abuse liability. *Journal of Consulting Clinical Psychology* 1993, 61:743–750.

7. Porchet HC, Benowitz NL, Sheiner LB: Pharmacodynamic model of tolerance: Application to nicotine. *Journal of Pharmacology and Experimental Therapeutics* 1988, 244:231–236.

8. Epstein LH, Caggiula AR, Perkins KA, McKenzie SJ, Smith JA: Conditioned tolerance to the heart rate effects of smoking. *Pharmacology, Biochemistry, and Behavior* 1991, 39:15–19.

9. Benowitz NL, Jacob P III, Jones RT, Rosenberg J: Interindividual variability in the metabolism and cardiovascular effects of nicotine in man. *Journal of Pharmacology and Experimental Therapeutics* 1982, 221:368–372.

10. Benowitz NL, Kuyt F, Jacob P III: Influence of nicotine on cardiovascular and hormonal effects of cigarette smoking. *Clinical Pharmacology and Therapeutics* 1984, 36:74–81.

11. Benowitz NL, Jacob P III: Intravenous nicotine replacement suppresses nicotine intake from cigarette smoking. *Journal of Pharmacology and Experimental Therapeutics* 1990, 254:1000–1005.

12. Benowitz NL, Jacob P III, Fong I, Gupta S: Nicotine metabolic profile in man: Comparison of cigarette smoking and transdermal nicotine. *Journal of Pharmacology and Experimental Therapeutics* 1994, 268:296–303.

13. Benowitz NL, Zevin S, Jacob P III: Sources of variability in nicotine and cotinine levels with use of nicotine nasal spray, transdermal nicotine, and cigarette smoking. *British Journal of Clinical Pharmacology* 1997, 43:259–267.

14. Zevin S, Jacob P III, Benowitz NL: Cotinine effects on nicotine metabolism. *Clinical Pharmacology and Therapeutics* 1997, 61:649–654.

15. Benowitz NL: Acute biological effects of nicotine and its metabolites. In Clarke, PBS, Quik M, Adlkofer F, Thurau K (eds): *Effects of Nicotine on Biological Systems II. Advances in Pharmacological Sciences.* Basel: Birkhauser Verlag, 1995, pp 9–16.

16. Benowitz NL, Fitzgerald GA, Wilson M, Zhang Q: Nicotine effects on eicosanoid formation and hemostatic function: Comparison of transdermal nicotine and cigarette smoking. *Journal of the American College of Cardiology* 1993, 22:1159–1167.

17. Benowitz NL: Nicotine and coronary heart disease. *Trends in Cardiovascular Medicine* 1991, 1:315–321.

Chapter **3**

Cardiovascular Toxicity of Nicotine in Animals

STEVE GOURLAY

Tobacco smoking is a well-known cause of cardiovascular diseases such as accelerated atherosclerosis, acute myocardial infarction, sudden cardiac death, stroke, and peripheral vascular occlusion.[1] However, the constituent of tobacco smoke that is responsible for long-term, adverse effects on the cardiovascular system is unknown. Potential candidates include carbon monoxide, nicotine, polycyclic hydrocarbons, and glycoproteins.

Acute administration of nicotine results in catecholamine release, and in healthy subjects this increases the heart rate, blood pressure, coronary blood flow, and myocardial oxygen demand. Although some tolerance to the sympathomimetic effects of nicotine develops during chronic administration,[2] the heart rate, daytime ambulatory systolic blood pressure, and urinary catecholamine excretion of regular smokers are higher than those of nonsmokers.[3,4] Furthermore, smokers have more blood pressure variability than nonsmokers, a fact consistent with the effects of intermittent nicotine dosing. It is unclear whether direct actions of nicotine on blood vessels, the myocardium, or platelets are relevant to human pathology.

Epidemiological studies of long-term treatment with pure nicotine have not been conducted. Relevant information can be inferred, however, from studies of nonsmoking users of chewing tobacco or snuff, who, like users of nicotine polacrilex gum, generally have levels of nicotine intake similar to those of smokers but minimal adverse changes in the cardiovascular risk-factor profile.[5,6] A well-conducted, prospective study of cardiovascular mortality associated with smoke-less tobacco use among Swedish construction workers indicated a level of risk inter-mediate between that of nonusers of tobacco and that of smokers.[7] However, its find-ings were not corroborated by a smaller, retrospective case–control study that found no excess risk of myocardial infarction among Swedish smokeless tobacco users.[8]

Assuming that nicotine contributes to long-term cardiovascular risk, one expla-nation for a lower risk level among smokeless tobacco users than smokers is that carbon monoxide and other products of tobacco combustion are partly responsi-ble for cardiovascular injury associated with cigarette smoking. Alternatively, nicotine delivered to the lungs by smoking (the fastest route of absorption, giving the highest peak plasma concentration) may be more harmful than slower absorp-tion achieved through the gastrointestinal tract, skin, or nasal mucosa, as occurs with users of smokeless tobacco or nicotine medications.

This chapter reviews the evidence regarding possible harmful effects of nico-tine, without the presence of other tobacco components, on atherosclerosis and myocardial ischemia available from research in animals. Since human experi-mentation in this area may often be impractical or unethical, evidence from ani-mal models is an important source of information.

Nicotine doses and pharmacokinetics

To study the toxicity of nicotine in cigarette smoke, experimental animals should have a similar route of nicotine absorption, plasma concentration, time relation-ship, and peak plasma concentration as nicotine derived from human smoking. In addition, research animals must have a pharmacodynamic response to nicotine similar to that of humans. Unfortunately, relatively high nicotine concentrations have been used to assess cardiovascular responses in most animal models re-ported to date, and it is unclear whether pharmacodyamic responses in research animals approximate human responses.

It is also difficult to mimic nicotine delivery by smoking without using smoke as a vehicle. Available nicotine aerosols do not deliver significant doses to the lower respiratory tract and, instead, deposit most of the drug in the upper airways, where absorption is slower.[9] Frequent, intermittent parenteral dosing is impracti-cal because many injections are required per day. Perhaps the closest model to smoking is that of the osmotic minipump, which delivers a constant infusion of nicotine for several weeks at a time. Osmotic minipumps are particularly suited to modeling effects of nicotine delivery from transdermal nicotine patches because of their similar pharmacokinetic profiles. Orally administered nicotine undergoes first-pass metabolism in the liver and gastrointestinal tract. As a result, plasma concentrations of nicotine are less predictable than with parenteral administra-tion, and the ratio of the plasma concentration of metabolites (particularly coti-nine) to nicotine is higher.[10] Nicotine's proximate metabolite, cotinine, has been reported to lower blood pressure in humans,[11] and to have cardiovascular effects in animals.[12,13] For these reasons, animal models using parenteral administration of nicotine are better suited to illustrate probable human effects.

Plasma concentrations of nicotine and cotinine vary considerably between subjects administered similar doses of nicotine; plasma concentrations must be measured to determine exposure and evaluate pharmacodynamic effects. In most of the in vivo studies, plasma concentrations of nicotine or cotinine were not measured. As a result, it is uncertain whether exposure to nicotine in these animals was comparable with that of humans. In general, the high per kilogram doses of nicotine that were used were expected to produce plasma nicotine concentrations that were much higher than those seen with human smoking.

In the few animal studies in which concentrations were measured, there was considerable interstudy variability. For example, in rats and guinea pigs, nicotine doses of 2 and 10 mg kg^{-1} day^{-1}, respectively, administered subcutaneously by osmotic minipumps produced plasma concentrations of 22–26 ng ml^{-1}, which is roughly equivalent to the levels achieved during human cigarette smoking.[14] Li et al.[15] reported that a much lower dose in rats, 0.5 mg kg^{-1}, most closely approximated human smoking. Doses of 5 mg kg^{-1} day^{-1} are often used in rats, but are reported to produce high plasma concentrations of nicotine, e.g., 651–1,489 ng ml^{-1} administered in drinking water[16] and 362 ng ml^{-1} administered by subcutaneous osmotic minipump.[15] Interspecies variability in nicotine metabolism has not been systematically studied.

Atherosclerosis

A review of long-term atherosclerosis experiments on nicotine and plasma lipoprotein concentrations, nicotine and vascular histopathology, and nicotine and calcium illustrates what has been learned from the few long-term, pathology-based studies of nicotine exposure published to date. This evidence sheds light on the mechanisms by which nicotine could contribute to atherosclerosis.

Long-term atherosclerosis experiments

Three published studies of chronic oral or subcutaneously administered nicotine treatment in nonsmoking rabbits failed to demonstrate increased atherosclerosis when the rabbits' diets lacked cholesterol.[17–19] The doses of nicotine varied from relatively low, 1 mg kg^{-1} day^{-1},[17] to high, 11 mg kg^{-1} day^{-1}.[18] The significance of these studies is doubtful, however, because it is unclear whether atherogenesis from exposure to cigarette smoke can be demonstrated in similar animal models without cholesterol feeding.

An increased rate of development of aortic[20] and carotid[18] atherosclerosis during intramuscular or subcutaneously administered nicotine treatment of cholesterol-fed rabbits suggests that nicotine may be atherogenic in the presence of hy-percholesterolemia. However, the rabbit atherosclerosis models are not readily generalizable to describe human outcomes, because the plasma concentrations of cholesterol produced were severalfold greater than the concentrations usually seen in hypercholesterolemic humans—there may be a threshold below which a synergistic effect of nicotine and hypercholesterolemia is no longer clinically rel-evant. In addition, high per kilogram (11 mg kg^{-1} day^{-1}) doses of nicotine were used in one study,[18] and plasma concentrations were not measured in either study. Fisher et al.[17] used a lower dose of subcutaneous nicotine (1 mg kg^{-1} day^{-1}) and a 2% cholesterol diet and failed to demonstrate increased atherosclerosis. A more realistic rabbit model, using a 3% cholesterol diet to mimic human plasma cho-lesterol concentrations, has demonstrated increased atherogenesis in response to environmental tobacco smoke exposure, but has not been used to study the effects of nicotine alone.[21] The findings of these studies suggest a potential causative role of nicotine in human atherosclerosis and warrant further investigation.

Nicotine and plasma lipoprotein concentrations

In rabbits or monkeys, chronic administration of nicotine alters blood lipoprotein levels toward a more atherogenic profile. Rabbits given nicotine 4 mg kg^{-1} day^{-1}, via subcutaneous minipump, and a 1% cholesterol diet develop higher low-den-sity lipoprotein (LDL) levels and lower high-density lipoprotein (HDL) levels than cholesterol-fed controls, without an increase in total cholesterol.[18] In another study, the total cholesterol level of rabbits given intramuscular nicotine, 3 mg kg^{-1} day^{-1}, and a 2% cholesterol diet was twice that of cholesterol-fed controls: 2,685 versus 1,140 mg dl^{-1}.[20] Similarly, LDL cholesterol was increased and HDL de-creased in monkeys given oral nicotine, 6 mg kg^{-1}, for 2 years.[22]

Cross-sectional studies in humans suggest that regular tobacco smoking pro-duces lipoprotein changes similar to those observed in animal studies of nicotine administration.[23,24] In contrast, studies of nicotine replacement products or smoke-less tobacco in humans show minimal adverse effects on the lipoprotein pro-file.[5,25,26] A recent study of 22 mg transdermal nicotine patch therapy, however, documented temporary inhibition of the normalization of HDL cholesterol and HDL$_2$ cholesterol levels after smoking cessation.[27] Thus, it appears likely that nicotine affects lipoprotein levels in an adverse manner. However, these effects may be concentration dependent and, as such, greater in cigarette smokers than in users of smokeless tobacco or nicotine replacement products—these effects would then be exaggerated by animal models using high-dose nicotine.

Nicotine and vascular histopathology

Deleterious morphological changes in rabbit and rodent endothelium are seen with chronic oral nicotine dosing of 2–5 mg kg^{-1} day^{-1}.[28,29] These effects include cytoplasmic vacuolation, mitochondrial swelling, subendothelial edema, development of microvilli, and cellular projections into the lumen. In addition, nicotine may increase endothelial permeability by altering the morphology of intercellular clefts.[29] In rats, nicotine at plasma concentrations relevant to humans is reported to increase myointimal thickening following mechanical endothelial injury[30] and alter aortic smooth muscle morphology from a contractile to a synthetic form.[31] Alteration of aortic smooth muscle morphology was concentration dependent, with lesser effects seen at concentrations of nicotine usually measured during human smoking. A dose–response effect of nicotine concentrations ranging from 10^{-9} to 10^{-5} M is reported for synthesis and polymerization of cytoskeleton in cultured vascular smooth muscle cells and, to a lesser extent, in endothelial cells.[32] Administration of oral flavonoids in rats has been reported to prevent endothelial injury resulting from single intravenous nicotine doses equivalent to one cigarette (≥ 12.5 μg kg^{-1}).[33]

Several indirect mechanisms may explain the vascular toxicity of nicotine. High doses of nicotine elevate plasma LDL cholesterol level and, thus, may indirectly promote endothelial damage.[34] An in vitro study of human hepatoma cells suggests that the effects of nicotine on hepatic lipoprotein formation are mediated indirectly via epinephrine.[35] By increasing the concentration of circulating epinephrine or its oxidation products, nicotine may promote cholesterol uptake in endothelial cells. This potentially atherogenic effect has been demonstrated in cultured human endothelium with supraphysiological concentrations of adrenochrome, an oxidation product of epinephrine and, to a lesser extent, with epinephrine itself.[36]

Direct toxicity of nicotine is suggested in studies of giant endothelial cell formation[37] and changes induced in cell cultures at nicotine concentrations relevant to human exposures and by nicotine's ability to increase intracellular calcium content in vitro, causing calcification of elastic fibers.[38]

It appears that indirect and direct mechanisms for endothelial cell injury can be ascribed to high-dose nicotine in animal models. Generalization of these models to human smoking or nicotine replacement treatment, where the plasma concentrations of nicotine and epinephrine are considerably lower than in most of the studies discussed, is uncertain.

Nicotine and calcium

The action of nicotine to increase the intracellular concentration of calcium may be relevant to atherogenesis. At neuronal cholinergic receptors, nicotine or acetylcholine binding opens calcium channels, resulting in a brief increase in intracellular calcium[39] and enhanced neural transmission. It is unknown whether similar receptors are present on endothelial or vascular smooth muscle cells and what their function might be. However, high concentrations of nicotine (10^{-4} M) increase intracellular calcium in cultured rat vascular smooth muscle cells.[38]

Calcium appears to have messenger and "killer" functions that could contribute to the development of atherosclerotic lesions.[38] Increased intracellular calcium is known to modulate several cellular systems, including protein kinase C, phospholipase C, and calmodulin. These enzyme systems can cause activation of ion channels, enhanced stimulation–secretion coupling, cytoskeletal rearrangement, and induction of transcription and translation of specific proteins.[40]

Such a cascade of events has been proposed as a model of endothelial cell, shear-force injury leading to atherosclerosis.[40] The messenger functions of intracellular calcium in vascular smooth muscle cells include vasoconstriction, migration, proliferation, and matrix production. Should the cell extrusion capacity for calcium be overcome, a cascade of intracellular events can lead to cell death and necrosis.

As a link in the atherosclerotic process, calcium is interesting because of the observation that in vivo atherogenic effects of various toxins, including nicotine, vitamin D, and oxidized LDL, can be inhibited by calcium channel-blocking drugs. Specifically, the ability of high-dose oral nicotine to cause early lesions in rat coronary arteries, with increased calcium content, has been inhibited by the concurrent administration of nifedipine.[38] Similar effects have been demonstrated in cultured rat coronary artery smooth muscle cells. In a vitamin D_3 and high-dose oral nicotine model of atherosclerosis, lesions develop very quickly.[38,41] Using this model, calcium antagonists are reported to prevent calcium accumulation and cell surface degeneration in endothelial cells of the aorta[42] and mesentery.[43] Nicotine, in oral doses of 2–5 mg kg^{-1} day^{-1}, has been shown to increase the calcium content of the aorta in rabbits, but without histological evidence of accelerated atherosclerosis.[19]

One explanation of the interaction of calcium channel-blocking drugs with the effects of nicotine is that the first step in the cascade of events could be attributable to nicotinic acetylcholine receptor activation. The calcium channel-blocking drug methoxyverapamil has been shown to decrease the calcium current through its action at this type of receptor.[44] The site of action could be local, at the endothelium or vascular smooth muscle, or in the adrenal gland, where secretion of catecholamines could be reduced. Alternatively, calcium antagonists may reduce the blood pressure of experimental animals, thereby reducing atherogenesis by an indirect mechanism. Studies of the effects of nicotine on arterial calcium homeostasis with chronic nicotine dosing at plasma concentrations equivalent to those seen with human smoking are needed to elucidate this area further.

Acute myocardial infarction and acute administration of nicotine

In dogs, intravenous nicotine in amounts equivalent to the dose from approximately five cigarettes in humans (80 μg kg^{-1}) exacerbates spontaneous cyclic reductions in coronary flow in an at-risk area of myocardium.[45] This was shown in a study by Folts and Bonebrake[45] in anesthetized dogs using mechanical, partial circumflex artery occlusion. Similar results were obtained with either cigarette smoke or intravenous nicotine. In 18 of the 21 dogs, occlusive events after exposure to smoke or nicotine were prevented by prior administration of the α-blocking drug phentolamine, suggesting that catecholamines mediated the response. The authors suggested that nicotine's effects were consistent with the formation of platelet thrombi in the coronary microcirulation, an effect they previously demonstrated in response to increased plasma catecholamine concentrations. This model implies a thrombotic mechanism, whereby nicotine could exacerbate ischemic myocardial damage in the setting of atherosclerotic plaque rupture, angioplasty, and other situations of endothelial damage.

A similar dose of intravenous nicotine, given 30 minutes before or 1 hour after temporary coronary occlusion, worsens myocardial dysfunction.[46] In a placebo-controlled experiment, transient ischemia was induced in dogs by 15 minutes of left anterior descending artery clamping. Segmental shortening recovered to only 29% of the preischemia baseline in nicotine-pretreated animals compared with 54% for saline-treated controls ($p < 0.01$). The dose of nicotine did not alter heart rate, blood pressure, or blood flow or cause myocyte necrosis. Interestingly, prior administration of N-2-mercaptoproprionyl glycine (MPG), a free-radical scavenging agent, prevented the effects of nicotine administration. The author hypothesized that nicotine may amplify oxidative ischemic injury.[46] It is unclear whether this effect could be due to the direct action of nicotine or to an indirect mechanism, such as increased concentrations of circulating catecholamines or local second messengers in the heart. Treatment with MPG in the absence of nicotine did not improve myocardial function.

Increased intracellular calcium accumulation is one mechanism by which nicotine may harm the myocardium during ischemia. During reperfusion, after global myocardial ischemia in isolated rat hearts, nicotine at a plasma concentration of 150 ng ml^{-1} has been shown to increase intracellular calcium compared with controls.[47] This effect was reduced by 3 days of pretreatment with the calcium channel blockers verapamil and anipamil.

Unfortunately, the findings with these animal models are not readily generalizable to the human situation, where nicotine is used chronically during smoking or nicotine replacement therapy. Substantial tolerance develops to nicotine's sympathomimetic cardiovascular effects during chronic nicotine intake,[2] and may lessen or cancel the ill effects demonstrated in nicotine-naive research animals. Nevertheless, since tolerance is not complete, bolus administration of nicotine in smoking or other rapid-delivery systems during chronic nicotine intake could conceivably affect the coronary circulation in the way that acute administration in nontolerant subjects does, although its effects would be less pronounced.

Acute myocardial infarction and chronic nicotine treatment

Unfortunately, the only studies of *chronic* nicotine treatment, more relevant to regular smoking or to the use of nicotine replacement therapy, used extremely high doses of nicotine (12 mg over 15 minutes intravenously per day in dogs), and it would be unwise to generalize these findings to humans. These studies reported increased myocardial infarct size after coronary artery ligation and promotion of early ventricular arrhythmias.[48,49] Animal studies with nicotine exposures closer to the usual human situation are needed to determine whether nicotine is a clinically significant cardiac toxin.

Conclusions

Animal experiments conducted to date indicate that nicotine may promote atherosclerosis, particularly when combined with hypercholesterolemia or endothelial injury. A case is made for increased intracellular concentration of calcium as a component of the mechanism of atherogenesis attributable to nicotine. Animal studies that model concentrations of nicotine seen during human smoking are needed to clarify the clinical importance of postulated atherogenic effects of nicotine. Studies comparing cigarette smoke exposure, nicotine, and placebo are needed to determine the relative importance of nicotine in smoking's atherogenic effects. Because it is fairly certain that smoking interacts with other risk factors, future testing should include challenge conditions and not just basic conditions.

Acute administration of high doses of nicotine can exacerbate myocardial ischemia caused by acute endothelial injury and occlusion of major coronary arteries in dogs. Further research is needed to examine whether chronic use of nicotine in doses relevant to human exposure can cause similar effects.

There are few data concerning the potentially differing effects of the rate of dosing of nicotine on the cardiovascular system. Nicotine delivered slowly results in lower peak arterial plasma levels than the same doses delivered rapidly and probably causes less adrenal release of catecholamines. Thus, nicotine from a transdermal nicotine patch may be less harmful than the same dose delivered by smoking. These facts should be considered when designing future animal models, as a slow-delivery method would be the best model of the effects of transdermal nicotine and a rapid-delivery method the best model of effects of nicotine from smoking.

Looking to the future, it will be interesting also to see if calcium channels and calcium channel blockers are relevant to the prevention or pathophysiology of smoking-related atherosclerosis. More long-term exposure experiments are needed in research animals with approximation of human plasma concentrations of nicotine.

References

1. U.S. Department of Health and Human Services: *Reducing the Health Consequences of Smoking: 25 Years of Progress.* A Report of the Surgeon General. Washington, DC: Government Printing Office, 1989.

2. Porchet HC, Benowitz NL, Sheiner LB: Pharmacodynamic model of tolerance: Application to nicotine. *Journal of Pharmacology and Experimental Therapeutics* 1988, 244:23–28.

3. Palatini P, Pessina AC, Graniero GR, Mormino P, Dorigatti F, Accurso V, et al.: The relationship between overweight, life style and casual and 24-hour blood pressures in a population of male subjects with mild hypertension: The results of the HARVEST study. *Giornal Italiano di Cardiolgia* 1995, 25:977–989.

4. Pickering T, Schwartz JE, James GD: Ambulatory blood pressure monitoring for evaluating the relationships between lifestyle, hypertension and cardiovascular risk. *Clinical and Experimental Pharmacology and Physiology* 1995, 22:226–231.

5. Allen SS, Hatsukami D, Jensen J, Grillo M, Bliss R: Effects of treatment on cardiovascular risk among smokeless tobacco users. *Preventive Medicine* 1995, 24: 357–362.

6. Eliasson M, Lundblad D, Hagg E: Cardiovascular risk factors in young snuff-users and cigarette smokers. *Journal of Internal Medicine* 1991, 230:17–22.

7. Bolinder G, Alfredsson L, Englund A, de Faire U: Smokeless tobacco use and increased cardiovascular mortality among Swedish construction workers. *American Journal of Public Health* 1994, 84:399–404.

8. Huhtasaari F, Asplund K, Stegmayr B, Wester PO: Tobacco and myocardial infarction: Is snuff less dangerous than cigarettes? *British Medical Journal* 1992, 305: 1252–1256.

9. Bergstrom M, Nordbert A, Lunell E, Antoni G, Langstrom B: Regional deposition of inhaled ^{11}C-nicotine vapor in the human airway as visualized by positron emission tomography. *Clinical Pharmacology and Therapeutics* 1995, 57:309–317.

10. Benowitz NL, Jacob III P, Savanapridi C: Determinants of nicotine intake while chewing nicotine polacrilex gum. *Clinical Pharmacology and Therapeutics* 1987, 41: 467–473.

11. Keenan RM, Hatsukami DK, Pentel PR, Thompson TN, Grillo MA: Pharmacodynamic effects of cotinine in abstinent cigarette smokers. *Clinical Pharmacology and Therapeutics* 1994, 55:581–590.

12. Dominiak P, Fuchs G, von Toth S, Grobecker H: Effects of nicotine and its major metabolites on blood pressure in anaesthetized rats. *Klinische Wochenschrift* 1985, 63:90–92.

13. Kuo B-S, Dryjski M, Bjornsson TD: Influence of nicotine and cotinine on the expression of plasminogen activator activity in bovine aortic endothelial cells. *Thrombosis and Haemostasis* 1989, 61:70–76.

14. Becker BF, Terres W, Kratzer M, Gerlach E: Blood platelet function after chronic treatment of rats and guinea pigs with nicotine. *Klinische Wochenschrift* 1988, 66 (suppl XI):28–36.

15. Li Z, Barrios V, Buchholz JN, Glenn TC, Duckles SP: Chronic nicotine administration does not affect peripheral vascular reactivity in the rat. *Journal of Pharmacology and Experimental Therapeutics* 1994, 271:1135–1142.

16. Lin S-J, Hong C-Y, Chang M-S, Chiang BN, Chien S: Long-term nicotine exposure increases aortic endothelial cell death and enhances transendothelial transport in rats. *Arteriosclerosis and Thrombosis* 1992, 12:1305–1312.

17. Fisher ER, Rothstein R, Wholey MH, Nelson R: Influence of nicotine on experimental atherosclerosis and its determinants. *Archives of Pathology* 1973, 96:298–304.

18. Strohschneider T, Oberhoff M, Hanke H, Hannekum A, Karsch KR: Effect of chronic nicotine delivery on the proliferation rate of endothelial and smooth muscle cells

in experimentally induced vascular wall plaques. *Clinical Investigation* 1994, 72: 908–912.

19. Schievelbien H, Londong V, Londong H, Grumbach H, Remplik V, Schauer A, et al.: Nicotine and arteriosclerosis. *Z Klin Chem* 1970, 8:190–196.

20. Stefanovich V, Gore I, Kahyama G, Iwanaga Y: The effect of nicotine on dietary atherogenesis in rabbits. *Experimental and Molecular Pathology* 1969, 11:71–81.

21. Zhu BQ, Sun YP, Sievers RE, Isenberg WM, Glantz SA, Parmley WW: Passive smoking increases experimental atherosclerosis in cholesterol-fed rabbits. *Journal of the American College of Cardiology* 1993, 21:225–232.

22. Cluette-Brown J, Mulligan J, Doyle K, Hagan S, Osmolski T, Hojnacki J: Oral nicotine induces an atherogenic lipoprotein profile. *Proceedings of the Society for Experimental Biology and Medicine* 1986, 182:409–413.

23. Craig WY, Palomaki GE, Haddow JE: Cigarette smoking and serum lipid and lipoprotein concentrations: An analysis of published data. *British Medical Journal* 1989, 298:784–788.

24. Freeman DJ, Griffin BA, Murray E, Lindsay GM, Gaffey D, Packard CJ, et al.: Smoking and plasma lipoproteins in man: Effects on low density lipoprotein cholesterol levels and high density lipoprotein subfraction distribution. *European Journal of Clinical Investigation* 1993, 23:630–640.

25. Allen SS, Hatsukami D, Gorsline J: Transdermal Nicotine Study Group. Cholesterol changes in smoking cessation using the transdermal nicotine system. *Preventive Medicine* 1994, 23:190–196.

26. Quensel M, Agardh C-D, Nilsson-Ehle P: Nicotine does not affect plasma lipoprotein concentrations in healthy men. *Scandanavian Journal of Clinical Laboratory Investigation* 1989, 49:149–153.

27. Biggerstaff KD, Moffat RJ, Martinez R: Influence of nicotine on the normalization of lipoprotein profiles. *Proceedings of the Second Annual Conference.* Washington, DC: Society for Research on Nicotine and Tobacco, 1996.

28. Booyse FM, Osikowicz G, Quarfoot AJ: Effects of chronic oral consumption of nicotine on rabbit aortic endothelium. *American Journal of Pathology* 1981, 102:229–238.

29. Zimmerman M, McGeachie J: The effect of nicotine on aortic endothelium: A quantitative ultrastructural study. *Atherosclerosis* 1987, 63:33–41.

30. Krupski WC, Olive GC, Weber CA, Rapp JH: Comparative effects of hypertension and nicotine on injury-induced myointimal thickening. *Surgery* 1987, 102:409–415.

31. Thyberg J: Effects of nicotine on phenotypic modulation and initiation of DNA synthesis in cultured arterial smooth muscle cells. *Virchows Archives [Cell Pathology]* 1986, 52:33–40.

32. Csonka E, Somogyi A, Augustin J, Haberbosch W, Schettler G, Jellinek H: The effect of nicotine on cultured cells of vascular origin. *Virchows Archives [Cell Pathology]* 1985, 407:441–447.

33. Hladovec J: Endothelial injury by nicotine and its prevention. *Experientia* 1978, 34: 1585–1586.

34. Campbell JH, Campbell JR: Cell biology of atherosclerosis. *Journal of Hypertension* 1994, 12(suppl):S129–S132.

35. Craig WY: The effect of compounds associated with cigarette smoking on the secretion of lipoprotein lipid by HepG2 cells. *Biochimica et Biophysica Acta* 1993, 1165:249–258.

36. Zhou Q, Hulea S, Kummerow FA: Effects of adrenochrome and epinephrine on human arterial endothelial cells in vitro. *Research Communications in Molecular Pathology and Pharmacology* 1995, 89:111–126.

37. Tulloss JH, Booyse FM: Effect of various agents and physical damage on giant cell formation in bovine aortic endothelial cell cultures. *Microvascular Research* 1978, 16:51–58.
38. Fleckstein-Grun G, Thimm F, Czirfuzs A, Matyas S, Frey M: Experimental vasoprotection by calcium antagonists against calcium-mediated arteriosclerotic alterations. *Journal of Cardiovascular Pharmacology* 1994, 24(suppl 2):S75–S84.
39. Gerber SH, Haunstetter A, Kruger C, Kaufmann A, Nobiling R, Haass M: Role of $[Na^+]_1$ and $[Ca^{2+}]_1$ in nicotine-induced norepinephrine release from bovine adrenal chromaffin cells. *American Journal of Physiology* 1995, 269(Cell Physiol 38): C572–C581.
40. Davies PF, Dull RO: How does the arterial endothelium sense flow? Hemodynamic forces and signal transduction. In Diana JN (ed): *Tobacco Smoking and Atherosclerosis.* New York: Plenum Press, 1990, pp 281–293.
41. Henrion D, Chillon J-M, Godeau G, Muller F, Capdeville-Atkinson C, Hoffman M, Atkinson J: The consequences of aortic calcium overload following vitamin D_3 plus nicotine treatment in young rats. *Journal of Hypertension* 1991, 9:919–926.
42. Higo K, Karasawa A, Kubo K: Protective effects of benidipine hydrochloride (KW-3049), a calcium antagonist, against experimental arterial calcinosis and endothelial dysfunction. *Journal of Pharmacobio-Dynamics* 1992, 15:113–120.
43. Henrion D, Chillon J-M, Capdeville-Atkinson C, Atkinson J: Effect of chronic treatment with the calcium channel blocker, isradipine, on vascular calcium overload produced by vitamin D_3 and nicotine in rats. *Journal of Pharmacology and Experimental Therapeutics* 1992, 260:1–8.
44. Boehm S, Huck S: Methoxyverapamil reduction of nicotine-induced catecholamine release involves inhibition of nicotinic acetylcholine receptor currents. *European Journal of Neuroscience* 1993, 5:1280–1286.
45. Folts JD, Bonebrake FC: The effects of cigarette smoke and nicotine on platelet thrombus formation in stenosed dog coronary arteries: Inhibition with phentolamine. *Circulation* 1982, 65:465–470.
46. Przyklenk K: Nicotine exacerbates postischemic contractile dysfunction of stunned myocardium in the canine model: Possible role of free radicals. *Circulation* 1994, 89: 1272–1281.
47. Panagiotopoulos S, Nayler WG: Nicotine-induced calcium overload during postischemic reperfusion. *Journal of Cardiovascular Pharmacology* 1987, 10:683–691.
48. Masden RR, Flowers NC: Extension of experimental infarction with nicotine and estimates of infarct size. *American Heart Journal* 1980, 99:342–348.
49. Sridharan MR, Flowers NC, Hand RC, Hand JW, Horan LG: Effect of various regimens of chronic and acute nicotine exposure on myocardial infarct size in the dog. *American Journal of Cardiology* 1985, 55:1407–1411.

Chapter 4

Cardiovascular Effects of Cigarette Smoke and Snuff

ÅKE WENNMALM

Nicotine has a variety of effects on the cardiovascular system.[1] Most, but not all, of these effects are based on increased sympathetic activity. Nicotine may facilitate sympathoadrenal activity by coupling to central cholinergic receptors or to sympathetic ganglia or by enhancing transmitter release at a given sympathetic impulse rate. Which of these effects is most important in people who self-administer nicotine is not entirely clear.

Enhanced sympathetic activity in the cardiovascular system manifests as tachycardia and hypertension. In the heart, increased sympathetic activity shortens the interval between the spontaneous depolarizations in the pacemaker cells in the atrial sinus node, thereby increasing the heart rate. There are also free sympathetic nerve endings in the ventricular myocardium. Increased discharge in these fibers will enhance myocardial contractility. Sympathetic stimulation of the heart then causes increased cardiac work, since the increased heart rate and contractility enhance the amount of blood pumped through the heart per time unit.

Sympathetic vasoconstrictor fibers in the vessel walls, particularly in the resistance vessels, innervate the smooth muscle layer in the wall of these vessels. Increased activity leads to α-adrenoceptor activation and subsequent vasoconstriction. The vasoconstriction, in turn, leads to enhanced systemic vascular resistance. The increased resistance results in increased blood pressure. Hence, the acute effects of nicotine in the cardiovascular system are tachycardia and hypertension.

Sympathetic nerves innervate fat tissue. Increased sympathetic activity produces lipolysis with elevated circulating levels of free fatty acids (FFA) and glycerol in the blood. Tissues like the myocardium and skeletal muscle extract various fuels required for their energy metabolism from the blood in proportion to their abundancies. Hence, increased plasma levels of FFA will increase FFA uptake in these tissues, thereby diverting the energy metabolism from carbohydrates to fat. Fat metabolism requires more oxygen per gram; therefore, increased sympathetic activity will have a distinct oxygen-demanding effect in that it will augment the amount of oxygen required for a given amount of energy to be produced. Via these mechanisms, nicotine has a dual effect on myocardial metabolism: It increases cardiac oxygen demand by increasing cardiac work and by elevating the amount of oxygen required for a given amount of cardiac work. Experimental studies in dogs have revealed that about half of the nicotine-induced rise in myocardial oxygen consumption is related to enhanced mechanical activity of the heart; the remaining rise is attributable to a metabolic stimulation of high FFA concentrations.[2]

Cardiovascular effects of cigarette smoke and nicotine in healthy subjects

It is well known that smoking elicits tachycardia and an increase in blood pressure. To study these events more systematically, Cryer et al.[3] recorded the effects of cigarette smoking, sham smoking, and smoking with and without sympathetic receptor blockade in 10 healthy subjects. They reported smoking-associated increments in plasma norepinephrine and epinephrine levels. They also observed elevated heart rate, blood pressure, plasma levels of glycerol, and lactate-to-pyruvate ratio, all of which were abolished by pretreatment with sympathetic receptor blockers. Sham smoking had no effect. Smoking elevated heart rates by 15–20 beats per minute and systolic and diastolic blood pressure by about 12 mm Hg. The peak effect was observed after about 10 minutes of smoking. Thereafter, heart rate and systemic blood pressure gradually dropped toward the presmoking level, which was reached after about 30 minutes. Plasma glycerol increased by almost 50%, and the lactate-to-pyruvate ratio almost doubled due to an increased plasma concentration of lactate and a decreased plasma concentration of pyruvate. The metabolic changes caused by cigarette smoking lasted longer than the cardiovascular effects.[3]

The metabolic effects of cigarette smoking were quantitatively addressed in a careful study by Hofstetter et al.[4] These authors assessed the effect of smoking on energy expenditure in eight healthy cigarette smokers who spent 24 hours in a metabolic chamber on two occasions: once without smoking and once with smoking 24 cigarettes per day. All other variables were kept constant. Smoking caused an increase in mean, 24-hour norepinephrine excretion of nearly 50% and increased total 24-hour energy expenditure by about 10%.

There is good reason to assume that both the cardiovascular and metabolic effects of smoking seen by Hofstetter et al.[4] were due to absorption of nicotine during smoking. In a later study, Benowitz et al.[5] compared the cardiovascular effects of cigarette smoke, smokeless tobacco (chewing tobacco and oral snuff), and nicotine gum. They reported that maximum levels of nicotine were similar with the different administration routes, but the overall nicotine exposure was higher after using smokeless tobacco because of the prolonged absorption. All types of tobacco administration studied increased heart rate and blood pressure. A tendency toward greater overall cardiovascular effects, however, was demonstrated with administration of smokeless tobacco.

Nicotine in a dose of 4 mg, administered to eight healthy nonsmoking men in chewing gum, was found to increase myocardial oxygen consumption more than had been expected from the increase in rate-pressure product.[6] Thus, the observed increases in heart rate (12 beats per minute) and mean arterial blood pressure (7 mm Hg) were paralleled by elevations in increased coronary flow and myocardial oxygen uptake (by about 20%), suggesting a direct metabolic effect of nicotine.

Effects of cigarette smoke and nicotine on platelet–vessel wall interaction in healthy subjects

Platelets play a key role in the hemostatic process. When a blood vessel is injured, platelets are activated to form a hemostatic plug that prevents blood loss via the injury. Platelet activation results in release of pro-aggregatory and -adhesive factors and also externalization of membrane glycoproteins that act as receptors for these ligands. Activated platelets rapidly form a hemostatic plug that completely occludes the blood vessel. Therefore, platelet activation is a potentially hazardous process requiring strict control, i.e., platelet activation must not occur in a normal, noninjured vessel. Thus, platelet activation requires external initiation by factors like thrombin, adenosine triphosphate, or collagen. Other mediators, like epinephrine, may facilitate aggregation or adhesion.

Endothelial factors, like prostacyclin (PGI_2) or nitric oxide, are continuously formed and secreted from the inner layer of the vessel wall to counteract platelet adhesion and aggregation. A delicate balance exists in a healthy, noninjured blood vessel between pro- and anti-aggregatory and -adhesive factors. This balance maintains platelet activity at a level at which adhesion and aggregation do not develop. However, if endothelial factors are eliminated, the balance shifts to a more pro-aggregatory and -adhesive state, requiring lower amounts of initiating factors (thrombin or collagen) to elicit formation of a platelet thrombus. Under such conditions, the platelet–vessel wall interaction is less sufficiently controlled, and the risk for platelet thrombus formation, with subsequent vascular occlusion, is increased.

Cigarette smoking is a commonly accepted risk factor for cardiovascular disease. Several small studies have indicated that cigarette smoking may enhance platelet formation of Thromboxane A_2 (TxA$_2$). To assess this in a defined population, a study was conducted in a random sample of Swedish men, aged 19–21 years, who were screened physically and mentally prior to entering military service.[7] Tobacco use habits were evaluated by a questionnaire, and a urinary sample was collected for analysis of TxA$_2$, the platelet pro-adhesive and -aggregatory prostanoid, and of PGI$_2$, its endothelial, anti-aggregatory counterpart. Urinary excretion of TxA$_2$ metabolite was higher in cigarette smokers than in those not using tobacco, and it correlated with daily cigarette consumption. Snuff users had no increase in their urinary excretion of TxA$_2$ metabolite, despite displaying urinary cotinine levels comparable with those of the cigarette smokers. The excretion of PGI$_2$ metabolite did not differ between nontobacco users, cigarette smokers, and snuff users. The conclusions from the study are that cigarette smoking, but not the use of snuff, facilitates the formation of TxA$_2$ and that this increased formation reflects platelet activation in the absence of vascular injury. Furthermore, it was concluded that such platelet activation may be of significance for subsequent development of cardiovascular disease.[7]

Recently, endothelial nitric oxide has been recognized as an important regulator of platelet function and vascular tone.[8] The continuous endothelial formation of nitric oxide throughout the vascular tree, maintains a steady degree of vascular relaxation. As a consequence, acute inhibition of endothelial nitric oxide formation results in hypertension. Endothelial nitric oxide also regulates platelet activity by counteracting both adhesiveness and aggregability. The effects of nitric oxide on vascular tone and platelet function are mediated via activation of soluble guanylate cyclase, which converts guanosine triphosphate to the second-messenger cyclic guanosine monophosphate. Loss of endothelial control of vascular tone and platelet function appears to develop in the presence of hypercholesterolemia, atherosclerosis, and diabetic angiopathy. The basis for endothelial dysfunction in these settings is probably not impaired formation, but rather increased degradation of nitric oxide.[9] It is generally accepted that the endothelial dysfunction in these disease states contributes to thromboembolism, vascular occlusion, and tissue infarction.

Celermajer et al.[10] used flow-mediated dilation of the brachial artery to evaluate endothelial dysfunction in various clinical conditions. They were able to demonstrate that flow-mediated, endothelium-dependent vasodilation was impaired or abolished in hypercholesterolemia and also in cigarette smokers without apparent vascular disease. The mechanism behind this important finding, which demonstrated that smoking has just as great a negative impact on endothelial function as advanced age, diabetes mellitus, atherosclerosis, or hypercholesterolemia, was not clear from their study.[10] Recently, experiments in isolated vessels yielded results indicating that cigarette smoking increases oxidative stress in the vessel wall,[11] thereby destroying nitric oxide in a manner closely resembling that occurring in the vessels in other disease states. Future studies will reveal whether this mechanism also is operative in vivo. However, it is clearly established that smoking has a negative effect on endothelial control of platelet activity and vascular tone. Such an inhibitory effect of cigarette smoking on endothelial function acts to reinforce the adverse effect of cigarette smoking on platelet TxA_2. Loss of endothelial nitric oxide shifts the balance between anti- and pro-thrombogenic factors acting at the platelet–vessel interface in a thrombogenic direction. Because the stimulatory effect of TxA_2 is also pro-thrombogenic, the smoking effects on TxA_2 and nitric oxide are expected to be additive, or possibly even synergistic.

Cigarette smoke and nicotine effects on platelet–vessel wall interaction in vascular disease

Nicotine seems to be a less hazardous agent of tobacco smoke in subjects without apparent cardiovascular disease. There is no doubt that cigarette smoking initiates and maintains events that can contribute to the development of atherosclerosis and its complications of thromboembolism and tissue infarction. However, it seems that nicotine administration is hardly more hazardous than subjecting a healthy person to seeing a horror movie. The risk related to the use of nicotine does, however, change when the drug is administered in subjects with atherosclerotic vascular disease. The basis for this may be that, in contrast to exercise, nicotine elicits sympathetic activation without a concomitant increase in organ blood flow. An isolated increase in sympathetic activity may tend to activate processes like vasoconstriction and platelet activation. If, in contrast, the sympathetic activation is elicited by physical exercise, the exercise will increase blood flow, enhancing endothelial nitric oxide formation. Thus, a new balance between pro- and anti-aggregatory forces takes place, and the risk for platelet thrombus formation is not altered.

Folts and Bonebrake[12] have developed an elegant model to study, in vivo, the effects of various interventions on coronary thrombogenicity. In open-chest dogs, an epicardial artery is made stenotic by an external occluder, limiting the cross-sectional area of the lumen. At a certain degree of occlusion, cyclic changes in coronary flow develop. These changes are abolished, or at least counteracted, by pretreatment of the animal with aspirin, prostacyclin, or nitroglycerin. Reductions in coronary flow are thought to represent formation of platelet thrombi at the site of occlusion; these platelet thrombi progressively diminish the cross-sectional area of the epicardial artery, limiting blood flow. Normalization of blood flow represents detachment of the thrombi and the subsequent washout caused by an increased flow rate in the remaining open lumen when the cross-sectional area is progressively decreased. The Folts model may, to some extent, reflect events occurring in humans with unstable angina. The recurring pain attacks are thought to reflect the formation of a platelet thrombus in a stenotic coronary vessel, leading to myocardial ischemia and angina. Pain relief is assumed to indicate washout of the platelet thrombus, with subsequent return of blood flow, ending the myocardial ischemia. Unstable angina is a condition that frequently leads to development of acute myocardial infarction. Progression of unstable angina into myocardial infarction is probably the consequence of a total coronary occlusion by a platelet thrombus, i.e., of a thrombus that is not washed away in the bloodstream. Factors that affect platelet thrombus formation at the site of a coronary stenosis are of great interest because they may protect against or promote the development of a complete occlusion.

The effect of nicotine on the cyclic flow reductions in the dog model have been studied.[12] Nicotine, administered intravenously in doses comparable with those achieved through absorption of cigarette smoke by the lungs, produced α-adrenergic stimulation and potentiation of platelet thrombus formation. Compared with controls, significant increases were observed with respect to the slope of the cyclic flow reductions, their number and their size, when nicotine was administered. The results may demonstrate a link between nicotine use and platelet thrombus formation.

A study showing the metabolic effects of nicotine in a state of ischemia in the myocardium was performed in open-chest dogs to assess the effect of nicotine given intravenously on the severity of myocardial ischemia following acute coronary artery occlusion.[13] Myocardial ischemia was recorded as the sum of ST elevations in epicardial electrocardiographic recordings from a number of sites. Administration of nicotine elevated the plasma levels of FFA and enhanced the sum of ST elevations significantly. When lipolysis was inhibited pharmacologically, nicotine failed to elevate the plasma levels of FFA or to augment the sum of ST elevations. The authors of this study concluded that increased severity of acute myocardial ischemic injury, induced by nicotine, probably was related to increased myocardial oxygen requirements caused by excess myocardial consumption of FFA.

Summary and conclusions

The effects of nicotine in the cardiovascular system are due to its sympathomimetic activity, which leads to heart rate acceleration, elevation of systolic and diastolic blood pressure, increased cardiac work (via increases in heart rate and myocardial contractility), and enhanced lipolysis. Cigarette smoking, in addition to causing the same effects as nicotine, enhances platelet formation of TxA_2 and inhibits endothelial formation of nitric oxide.

The most serious pharmacological effects of cigarette smoking—from a cardiovascular point of view—are enhanced platelet formation of TxA_2 and inhibited endothelial formation of nitric oxide. These effects shift platelet–vessel wall interaction in a pro-thrombogenic direction, thereby promoting vascular occlu-sion and tissue infarction. The pro-thrombogenic activity of cigarette smoking is not due to its content of nicotine—nicotine does not seem to have such an effect.

References

1. Benowitz NL: Pharmacologic aspects of cigarette smoking and nicotine addiction. *New England Journal of Medicine* 1988, 319:1318–1330.
2. Mjös OD, Ilebekk A: Effects of nicotine on myocardial metabolism and performance in dogs. *Scandinavian Journal of Clinical and Laboratory Investigation* 1973, 32: 75–80.
3. Cryer PE, Haymond MW, et al.: Norepinephrine and epinephrine release and adrener-gic mediation of smoking-associated hemodynamic and metabolic events. *New Eng-land Journal of Medicine* 1976, 295:573–577.
4. Hofstetter A, Schutz Y, et al.: Increased 24-hour energy expenditure in cigarette smok-ers. *New England Journal of Medicine* 1986, 314:79–82.
5. Benowitz NL, Porchet H, et al.: Nicotine absorption and cardiovascular effects with smokeless tobacco use: Comparison with cigarettes and nicotine gum. *Clinical Phar-macology and Therapy* 1988, 44:23–28.
6. Kaijser L, Berglund B: Effect of nicotine on coronary blood-flow in man. *Clinical Physiology* 1985, 5:541–552.
7. Wennmalm Å, Benthin G, et al.: Relation between tobacco use and urinary excretion of thromboxane A_2 and prostacyclin metabolites in young men. *Circulation* 1991, 83: 1698–1704.
8. Moncada S, Palmer RMJ, et al.: Nitric oxide: physiology, pathophysiology, and phar-macology. *Pharmacological Reviews* 1991, 43:109–142.
9. Wennmalm Å: Nitric oxide (NO) in the cardiovascular system—Role in atherosclero-sis and hypercholesterolemia. *Blood Pressure* 1994, 3:279–282.
10. Celermajer DS, Sorensen KE, et al.: Non-invasive detection of endothelial dysfunc-tion in children and adults at risk of atherosclerosis. *Lancet* 1992, 340:1111–1115.
11. Raij L, Nagy J, et al.: Mechanisms of cigarette smoke induced impairment of endothe-lium dependent modulation of vascular tone. *Circulation* 1994, 90:I-575.
12. Folts JD, Bonebrake FC: The effects of cigarette smoke and nicotine on platelet thrombus formation in stenosed dog coronary arteries: Inhibition with phentolamine. *Circulation* 1982, 65:465–470.
13. Ilebekk A, Mjös OD: Effect of nicotine on severity of acute myocardial ischemic injury in dogs. *Scandinavian Journal of Clinical and Laboratory Investigation* 1974, 33:145–151.

Chapter **5**

Toxicity of Nicotine Replacement in Patients with Coronary Artery Disease

STEPHEN I. RENNARD, DAVID DAUGHTON,
and JOHN WINDLE

Both cigarette smoking and nicotine are known to have a number of cardiovascular effects. Specifically, smoking can increase heart rate and acutely increase blood pressure[1-4]; nicotine can produce similar effects.[5-7] These effects should increase myocardial oxygen demand. In addition, smoking may induce coronary vasoconstriction in the presence of coronary artery disease.[8,9] Nicotine itself may also decrease coronary blood flow, perhaps by activating an α-adrenergic–mediated process.[10,11] Taken together, these effects could impair myocardial oxygen delivery and lead to symptoms in smokers with coronary artery disease. Since coronary artery disease might be relatively common in smokers, such toxicity could be important clinically during nicotine replacement therapy. To help address this question, three studies have been conducted specifically to assess cardiac toxicity in individuals with coronary artery disease.

Working group for the study of transdermal nicotine

A total of 156 subjects with documented coronary artery disease were enrolled.[12] Coronary artery disease was established if there was a documented history of myocardial infarction, a prior angioplasty or coronary artery bypass surgery for coronary artery disease, an abnormal coronary artery angiogram documenting at least 60% obstruction of a major vessel, or classic angina together with either an abnormal exercise test or an abnormal nuclear scan. Importantly, other conditions were required to be stable, including cardiac disease. That is, no patients were enrolled with unstable angina, with serious unsuccessfully treated arrhythmias, with vascular spasm, with recent (within 3 months) myocardial infarction, or with hemodynamically significant valvular disease.

The study was a prospective, double-blind, randomized trial in which subjects were randomized to receive either active (14 mg/day) transdermal nicotine or placebo patches. After 1 week, subjects could opt to use a larger active (21 mg/day) or placebo patch. In addition, all subjects received a behavioral support program that included a 45–60-minute weekly group program of 5–15 patients per group. The support program sessions were conducted by trained counselors who reviewed individual subject progress and provided behavioral therapy aimed at both cessation and prevention of relapse. No financial incentive for quitting was required. There were no telephone contacts or buddy systems used. Of the 156 subjects, two were spouses and one was excluded randomly for analysis, resulting in 155 evaluable subjects.

At the end of the 5-week treatment period, 36% of the active treatment subjects and 22% of the placebo subjects were abstinent, defined as no smoking during the last 4 weeks and an expired carbon monoxide level of less than 8 parts per million ($p < 0.05$).

Eleven subjects dropped from the study; 3 were receiving active patch and 8 were receiving placebo. Reasons for termination are summarized in Table 5-1. A number of specific cardiovascular safety evaluations were performed. There were no deaths or acute myocardial infarctions in either group during the study period. There was a trend toward a decrease in angina frequency in both groups, but no difference in angina frequency was observed between the placebo and treatment groups. Similarly, no difference between the placebo and the active group was reported for palpitations, dyspnea, nausea, dizziness, insomnia, or rash. A number of electrocardiographic features were measured with routine

Table 5-1. Reasons for patch discontinuation*

Placebo ($n = 8$)	Active ($n = 3$)
Angina (3)	Chest pain
Hospitalization (2)†	Nausea (2)
Electrocardiographic	Palpitations
Syncope	Stress
Diarrhea	
Skin Rash	
Paresthesia	
Palpitation	

*Prevalence of each symptom was in one subject unless otherwise indicated; several subjects experienced multiple symptoms.
†One subject was hospitalized for chest pain and underwent bypass surgery; another for ataxia, vomiting, diarrhea, and dizziness on target quit day, attributed to nicotine withdrawal.

electrocardiograms and with Holter monitors. (Holter monitors were performed at only one of the four study sites.) No differences were observed between the placebo and the treatment group for any electrocardiographic or Holter monitor features.

In summary, this study in 155 subjects treated with transdermal nicotine patch for 5 weeks demonstrated a statistically significant improvement in smoking quit rate without demonstrating any change in the incidence of toxic events.[12]

The available data, however, have several important limitations. First, patients were studied when their disease was stable. The safety of nicotine replacement in the setting of an acute coronary event, therefore, was not tested. Second, patients with evidence of coronary artery spasm were excluded. As cigarette smoking has been reported to increase vasospastic angina,[13,14] the safety of nicotine in this setting is also not established. The dose of nicotine used in the majority of patients, moreover, was moderate (14 mg/day), and the effect of nicotine at higher doses was not assessed. Third, the event rate observed for myocardial infarctions was very low. An increase in infarctions at a rate too low to be observed, therefore, is also not excluded.

Joseph Veterans' Administration study

In the Joseph Veterans' Administration study, 584 veterans or their dependents with a history of cardiovascular disease were enrolled.[15] Subjects had to have one or more of history of myocardial infarction, history of coronary bypass surgery or angioplasty, stenosis of at least 50% in at least on major coronary artery as seen with coronary angiography, or a clinical history of angina, congestive heart failure, cor pulmonale, arrhythmia, peripheral vascular disease, or cerebrovascular disease. Exclusions included unstable angina or myocardial infarction, coronary artery bypass surgery, angioplasty, or hospitalization for cardiac arrhythmias within 2 weeks before randomization.

The study subjects received a 10-week course of transdermal nicotine (beginning at 21 mg/day and tapering to 7 mg/day) or placebo. At 14 weeks, after randomization, 21% of subjects receiving nicotine patch and 9% of subjects on placebo patch were continuing to abstain from smoking. The primary endpoints for the study included death, myocardial infarction, cardiac arrest, and hospitalization due to increased severity of angina, arrhythmias, or congestive heart failure. The incidence of primary endpoints was 5.4% with nicotine treatment and 7.9% with placebo. Secondary endpoints included hospital admission for peripheral vascular disease, cerebrovascular disease, or other reasons and outpatient visits for increased severity of atherosclerotic cardiovascular disease. Secondary endpoints occurred in 11.9% of subjects on nicotine patch and 9.7% on placebo. Thus, this study, as did the previous study, found no evidence that nicotine replacement therapy aggravates cardiovascular disease.

Mahmarian study

Mahmarian and coworkers[16] studied 31 smokers with known coronary heart disease and significant myocardial perfusion defects on baseline exercise thallium SPECT testing. Subjects were treated with 14- and 21-mg patches, each for a minimum of 3 days. Following each dose of nicotine, the exercise thallium SPECT study was repeated. Most of the subjects continued to smoke while on nicotine patch treatment.

Despite significantly greater plasma nicotine concentrations while using nicotine patches (owing to combined patch use and cigarette smoking), the reversible myocardial perfusion defect size was smaller during nicotine patch therapy compared with baseline while smoking without patches. The carbon monoxide levels were lower despite smoking while on the patches because subjects smoked fewer cigarettes. The reduction in the perfusion defect size on thallium scan correlated most closely with the reduction in carbon monoxide level. Thus, despite higher plasma nicotine concentrations, the extent of myocardial perfusion defects, which predicts later acute cardiovascular events, was improved. This study suggests that it is most likely that carbon monoxide or other combustion products rather than nicotine are responsible for aggravation of myocardial ischemia that is produced by cigarette smoking

Summary and conclusions

Potential cardiac toxicity has achieved some notoriety due to reports in the news media of clusters of myocardial infarctions among patients who use the nicotine patch and smoke.[17] These issues attracted sufficient attention to require special FDA Food and Drug Administration.[18] Shortly after the introduction of the patch, this question was assessed. At that time, approximately 3 million prescriptions for the patch had been made with an average use of 6 weeks per prescription. Estimating the myocardial infarction rate as 6 per 1,000 patient-years among smokers, an expected number of myocardial infarctions would be approximately 2,250. To that date, only 33 events had been reported. The reported cases, therefore, certainly do not support an increased incidence of toxicity among smokers. Such an analysis, obviously, makes a number of assumptions. Nevertheless, both the available clinical trial and the clinical experience reported to date are consistent with the relative safety of transdermal nicotine in stable patients with cardiac disease. Considering that smokers are at increased risk for myocardial infarction and that smoking cessation can reduce that risk substantially and significantly, transdermal nicotine in such patients would currently be regarded as an appropriate therapeutic option.

References

1. Cellina GU, Honour AJ, Littler WA: Direct arterial pressure, heart rate and electrocardiogram during cigarette smoking in unrestricted patients. *American Heart Journal* 1975, 89:18–25.
2. Groppelli A, Giorgi DMA, Omboni S, Parati G, Mancia G: Persistent blood pressure increase induced by heavy smoking. *Journal of Hypertension* 1992, 10:495–499.
3. Beere PA, Glagov S, Zarins CK: Retarding effect of lowered heart rate on coronary atherosclerosis. *Science* 1984, 226:180–182.
4. Benowitz NL, Kuyt F, Jacob P: Influence of nicotine on cardiovascular and hormonal effects of cigarette smoking. *Clinical Pharmacology and Therapeutics* 1984, 36: 74–81.
5. Benowitz NL, Porchet H, Sheiner L, Jacob P: Nicotine absorption and cardiovascular effects with smokeless tobacco use: comparison with cigarettes and nicotine gum. *Clinical Pharmacology and Therapeutics* 1988, 44:23–28.
6. Benowitz NL, Peyton J, Jones RT, Rosenberg J: Interindividual variability in the metabolism and cardiovascular effects of nicotine in man. *Journal of Pharmacology and Experimental Therapeutics* 1982, 221:368–372.
7. Sutherland G, Russell MAH, Stapleton J, Feyerabend C, Ferno O: Nasal nicotine spray: A rapid nicotine delivery system. *Psychopharmacology* 1992, 108:512–518.
8. Klein LW, Ambrose J, Pichard A, Holt J, Gorlin R, Teichholz LE: Acute coronary hemodynamic response to cigarette smoking in patients with coronary artery disease. *Journal of the American College of Cardiology* 1984, 3:879–886.
9. Nicod P, Rehr R, Winniford MD, Campbell WB, Firth BG, Hillis LD: Acute systemic and coronary hemodynamic and serologic responses to cigarette smoking in long-term smokers with atherosclerotic coronary artery disease. *Journal of the American College of Cardiology* 1984, 4:964–971.
10. Woodman OL: Coronary vascular responses to nicotine in the anaesthetized dog. *Naunyn Schmiedebergs Archives of Pharmacology* 1991, 343:65–69.
11. Kaijser L, Berglund B: Effect of nicotine on coronary blood-flow in man. *Clinical Physiology* 1985, 5:541–552.
12. Working Group for the Study of Transdermal Nicotine in Patients with Coronary Artery Disease: Nicotine replacement therapy for patients with coronary artery disease. *Archives of Internal Medicine* 1994, 154:989–995.
13. Raymond R, Lynch J, Underwood D, Leatherman A, Mehdi R: Myocardial infarction and normal coronary arteriography: A 10 year clinical and risk analysis of 74 patients. *Journal of the American College of Cardiology* 1988, 11:471–477.
14. Caralis DG, Ubeydullah D, Kern MJ, Cohen JD: Smoking is a risk factor for coronary spasm in young women. *Circulation* 1992, 85:905–909.
15. Joseph AM, Norman SM, Ferry LH, Prochazka AV, Westman EC, Steele BG, Sherman SE, Cleveland M, Antonnucio DO, Hartman N, McGovern PG: The safety of transdermal nicotine as an aid to smoking cessation in patients with cardiac disease. *New England Journal of Medicine* 1996, 335:1792–1798.
16. Mahmarian JJ, Moye LA, Nasser GA, et al.: Nicotine patch therapy in smoking cessation reduces the extent of exercise-induced myocardial ischemia. *Journal of the American College of Cardiology* 1997, 30:125–130.
17. Hwang SL, Waldholz M: Heart attacks reported in patch users still smoking. *Wall Street Journal* June 19, 1992:B1.
18. United States Food and Drug Administration: Transcript of the 23rd meeting of the Drug Abuse Advisory Committee, Rockville, MD: July 14, 1992.

Part II

Nicotine and Cancer

Tobacco use is a major preventable cause of cancer in developed countries. It is estimated that 30% of cancers can be attributed to tobacco use. Many tobacco-induced cancers appear at anatomical sites of direct exposure to tobacco or tobacco smoke, such as the lungs, mouth, and esophagus. However, other tobacco-related cancers occurring away from the direct site of exposure, such as cancers of the bladder, pancreas, and liver, as well as leukemia, suggesting that tobacco use produces systemic exposure to carcinogens.

Naturally, the possibility that nicotine might contribute to carcinogenesis must be considered. While there is no evidence that nicotine itself causes cancer in humans, understanding possible mechanisms by which nicotine could contribute to carcinogenesis is important. The role nicotine could play in cancer is reviewed in Part II. Topics include the metabolism of nicotine to reactive intermediates that bind to macromolecules, the nitrosation of nicotine and related alkaloids to form carcinogenic nitrosamines, and neuroendocrine modulation of cancer. The research presented in Part II is important in helping investigators to design future studies on the safety of nicotine administered for long periods of time.

Chapter **6**

Studies on the Metabolic Fate of (S)-Nicotine and Its Pyrrolic Analog β-Nicotyrine

NEAL CASTAGNOLI, JR., XIN LIU,
MARK K. SHIGENAGA, RICHARD WARDROP,
and KAY CASTAGNOLI

This chapter discusses the possibility that nicotine, and/or some of the minor tobacco alkaloids, may be biotransformed to chemically reactive intermediates that, following chronic exposure, could give rise to health hazards, including cancer. It will be useful to define the metabolic profile of (S)-nicotine in order to identify possible chemical links to the biological properties of this important component. This chapter examines the pathways responsible for these conversions and the metabolic fate of the cyclic tertiary amine (S)-nicotine (**1**) and its pyrrolic analog β-nicotyrine (**2**) (Fig. 6-1), with particular emphasis on the possible formation of chemically reactive metabolites that may contribute to the adverse health outcomes associated with chronic tobacco use.

The oxidative metabolism of the tobacco alkaloid (S)-nicotine leads to 3-(R)-hydroxy-5-(S)-cotinine (*trans*-3-hydroxycotinine) as the principal urinary metabolite. The pathway responsible for the formation of this product initially involves cytochrome P450–catalyzed oxidation of (S)-nicotine to yield the corresponding 1,5-iminium intermediate, which is further oxidized in a reaction catalyzed by liver aldehyde oxidase to yield the pyrrolidinone (S)-cotinine, the precursor to *trans*-3-hydroxycotinine. In tissues that do not contain aldehyde oxidase, the intermediate iminium ion can be converted to the pyrrolic product β-nicotyrine. Because of β-nicotyrine's potential to undergo bioactivation to reactive metabolites that may contribute to the toxicity associated with chronic exposure to tobacco products, researchers have undertaken in vitro and in vivo

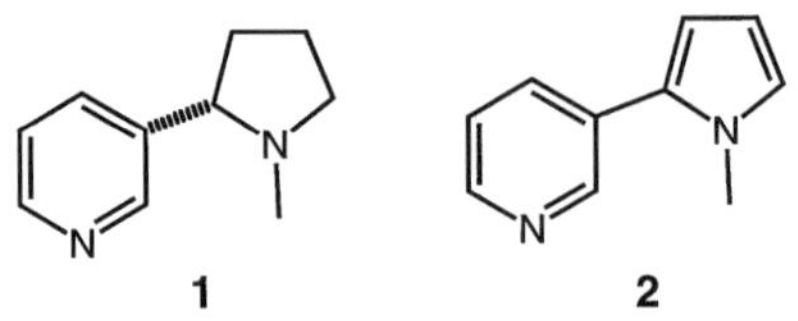

Figure 6-1. Structures of (S)-nicotine (1) and β-nicotyrine (2).

studies of its metabolic fate. A combination of high performance liquid chromatography (HPLC)–diode array, HPLC–mass spectrometry (MS), and gas chromatography (GC-MS)—analytical methodologies with synthetic efforts has provided evidence that this compound undergoes initial epoxidation to form an arene oxide that rearranges to a highly unstable mixture of tautomeric species that includes 2-hydroxy-1-methyl-5-(3-pyridyl)pyrrole. Autoxidation of this compound in vitro results in the generation of the 5-hydroxypyrrolinone derivative. In vivo, however, this 5-hydroxypyrrole derivative suffers an alternative fate that leads to the formation of *cis*-3-hydroxycotinine, that is, the diastereoisomer of *trans*-3-hydroxycotinine, the major urinary metabolite of (S)-nicotine.

Catalysts for the biotransformation of tertiary amines

The most important catalysts for the biotransformation of tertiary amines are members of the cytochrome P450 family of hemoproteins, which catalyze the 2-electron oxidation of the amine substrate (3) to form the corresponding iminium oxidation product (7).[1] The generally, but not universally,[2] accepted catalytic pathway (Fig. 6-2)[3] assumes an initial, single-electron transfer step from the substrate nitrogen lone pair to the P450-generated perferryl oxygen species (Fe^{V}O), leading to an aminyl radical cation 4, which, following loss of an acidic α-proton, forms an intermediate, carbon-centered radical 5. Radical recombination between 5 and Fe^{V}OH yields the carbinolamine 6, which will be in equilibrium with 7, and eventually undergoes hydrolysis to form the aldehyde 8 and dealkylated amine 9.

The substrate molecules in these transformations undergo a net oxidative N-dealkylation reaction. Cyclic tertiary amines (10) also undergo oxidative N-

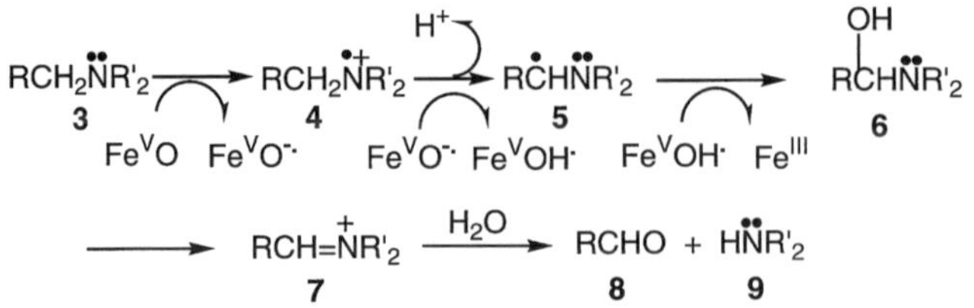

Figure 6-2. Pathway for the cytochrome P450-catalyzed oxidations of tertiary amines.

dealkylation via hydrolysis of the enzyme-generated exocyclic iminium interme-diates **11** to yield aldehydes **8** and the cyclic secondary amines **12** (Fig. 6-3). The corresponding oxidation of a ring α-carbon atom generates the cyclic iminium in-termediate **13.** Unlike the exocyclic regioisomer **11,** hydrolytic cleavage of **13** to yield the aminoaldehyde **14** is a reversible reaction, and, consequently, the fate of **13** must be considered separately. Often, these intermediary metabolites are oxi-dized further to the corresponding lactam **15** in a reaction that is catalyzed by the liver cytosolic enzyme aldehyde oxidase.[4]

(S)-Nicotine (**1**) is a cyclic tertiary amine that undergoes α-carbon oxidation (Scheme 6-4) at C-5 of the pyrrolidine ring in a reaction catalyzed by cytochrome P450 to form the corresponding iminium intermediate **16.**[5] In the presence of aldehyde oxidase, the iminium intermediate is rapidly converted to the lactam (S)-cotinine (**17**), the principal circulating metabolite of (S)-nicotine.[6] Subse-quently, **17** is oxidized further to *trans*-3-hydroxycotinine (**18**), the principal uri-nary metabolite of (S)-nicotine.[7] Aldehyde oxidase appears to be localized in liver tissue, and, consequently, the iminium intermediate generated in extrahepatic tis-sues might undergo alternative biotransformations from those observed in the liver. Since iminium species such as **16** are strong electrophiles that react with nu-cleophilic groups, researchers entertained the possibility that, in the absence of liver cytosolic aldehyde oxidase, the cytochrome P450-catalyzed oxidation of (S)-nicotine could produce **16,** or other reactive metabolites, that might form co-valent bonds with macromolecules. Such covalent association with macromole-cules is consistent with older literature reports describing the long retention of ^{14}C label in the respiratory tract of rodents treated with [14]C-(S)-nicotine.[8,9] Also consistent with the lung as a potential target for (S)-nicotine metabolite-mediated toxicities is the efficiency with which lung P450 catalyzes the oxidation of (S)-nicotine; estimates of turnover numbers at 100 μM substrate are 1.7 min^{-1} for liver P450 and 6.33 min^{-1} for lung P450.[10]

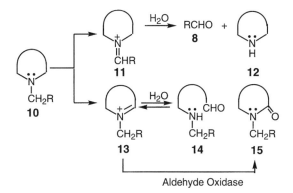

Aldehyde Oxidase

Figure 6-3. Alternative oxidative biotransformation pathways for cyclic tertiary amines.

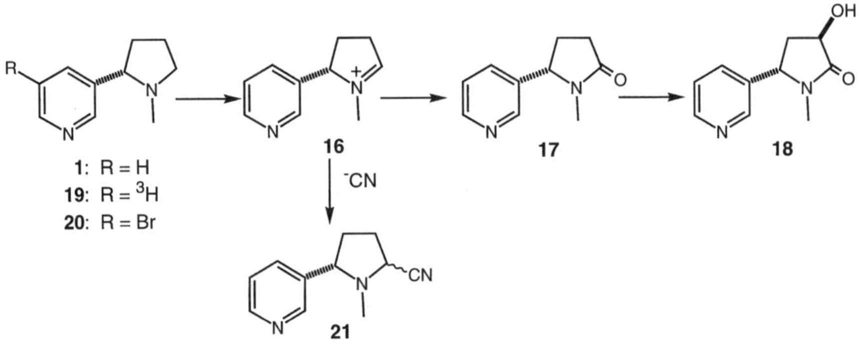

Figure 6-4. Metabolic fate of (S)-nicotine (**1**).

Possible formation of reactive metabolites from (S)-nicotine

To evaluate the possible formation of reactive metabolites from (S)-nicotine, researchers synthesized carrier-free (S)-nicotine-5-^{3}H (**19**) by tritiolysis of (S)-5-bromonicotine (**20**).[11] When incubated with rabbit liver microsomal preparations in the absence of NADPH, the starting amine was recovered fully, and no evidence of covalent association with the macromolecular fraction of the incubation mixture was evident. In the presence of NADPH, on the other hand, a time-dependent labeling of the microsomal protein was observed (Fig. 6-5).[12] Furthermore, the amount of substrate metabolized closely paralleled the amount of label incorporated into the microsomal protein. The partition ratios—(S)-nicotine metabolized per (S)-nicotine equivalents covalently bound—were estimated to be 470 for rabbit liver microsomes and 230 for rabbit lung microsomes. In addition to the NADPH dependence, researchers found that the extent of inhibition of (S)-nicotine metabolism by various agents such as SKF 525-A paralleled the incorporation of label into microsomal protein. Consequently, it is clear that this molecule undergoes bioactivation to reactive species that can form covalent adducts with microsomal proteins.

In view of these results, researchers have attempted to characterize the metabolic profile of (S)-nicotine in terms of the formation of reactive and potentially toxic metabolites. Of particular interest was the possibility that the iminium ion **16** may undergo covalent bond formation with nucleophilic functionalities on microsomal proteins. Based on earlier results,[13] researchers anticipated that it would be possible to intercept the iminium ion with cyanide to form the corresponding cyano adduct **21**. However, NaCN was found to inhibit the rate of metabolism of (S)-nicotine and the binding of radioactivity to microsomal protein to the same

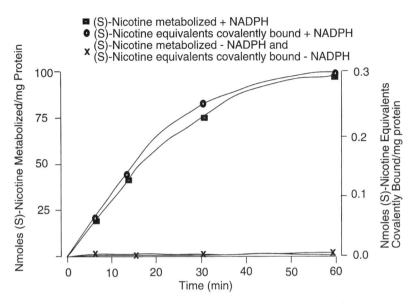

Figure 6-5. Metabolism-dependent covalent binding of (S)-nicotine-5[3]H to liver microsomal protein.

extent, suggesting that the iminium ion itself may not be involved in covalent binding.

A consideration of the structure of the iminium ion **16** and the known mono-amine oxidase B (MAO-B) substrate properties of various unsaturated cyclic tertiary amines[14,15] led researchers to examine the interactions of **16** with beef liver MAO-B.[10] The time-dependent and enzyme concentration–dependent formation of a single metabolite was observed by HPLC. Preincubation with pargyline, an MAO-B inactivator, blocked formation of the metabolite, confirming the catalytic role of the enzyme. Diode array analysis established the λ_{max} of this metabolite as 284 nm, identical to that of the pyrrolic tobacco alkaloid β-nicotyrine.[2] It was possible to confirm this assignment by comparing the GC-electron impact (EI) mass spectrum of the HPLC-purified metabolite with that of synthetic **2**. In separate experiments involving rabbit lung microsomal incubation mixtures and tritium-labeled (S)-nicotine, the formation of an NADPH-dependent radioactive peak with λ_{max} 286 nm was observed in the HPLC chromatogram with a slightly different retention time from that of synthetic **2**. Although full characterization of this metabolite remains to be accomplished, it is reasonable to suspect that it is either β-nicotyrine or a closely related molecule. Consequently, smokers are likely to be exposed to low levels of β-nicotyrine.

Metabolic fate of pyrrolic or related five-member nitrogen heterocyclic systems

Relatively little is known about the metabolic fate of pyrrolic or related five-membered nitrogen heterocyclic systems. It was expected, however, that the electron-rich pyrrolic moiety of β-nicotyrine would be susceptible to cytochrome P450–catalyzed oxidation and anticipated that the resulting metabolites would be chemically unstable and could contribute to the covalent binding of (S)-nicotine to biomacromolecules. Therefore, researchers examined the metabolism of β-nicotyrine both in vitro and in vivo.[16]

Turnover estimates of 7.9 min^{-1} for rabbit lung P450 and 2 min^{-1} for rabbit liver P450 confirmed the expectation that β-nicotyrine would be a good substrate for the cytochrome P450 monooxygenases.[10] HPLC–diode array and spectroscopic analyses, coupled with comparisons of synthetic standards, led to the characterization of the P450-generated equilibrium mixture of the 3- and 4-pyrrolinones (25 and 24, respectively).[17] The formation of these pyrrolinones probably proceeds via the reaction sequence summarized in Figure 6-6. Initial cytochrome P450–catalyzed oxidation of the electron-rich pyrrole moiety generates the unstable epoxide 22, which will be in equilibrium with the 5-hydroxypyrrole (23) and the two tautomeric pyrrolinones 24 and 25.

In the presence of O$_2$, the pyrrolinones 24 and 25 undergo spontaneous autoxidation. Two products are formed, but only one is chemically stable. The stable, late-appearing autoxidation product has been characterized as the 5-hydroxy-3-pyrrolinone derivative 29, which is probably generated by the pathway summarized in Figure 6-7. Liquid chromotography-chemical ionization LC-CI mass spectral analysis established that the unstable, early-appearing autoxidation product is isomeric with 29, which may be the corresponding 3-hydroxy-4-pyrrolinone 30 rearranging to the more stable and later-appearing 29. The postulated pathway leading to these products is summarized in Figure 6-7. Initial transfer of

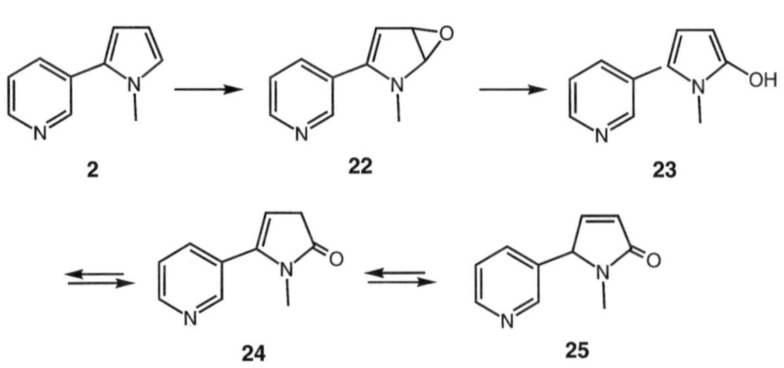

Figure 6-6. Proposed metabolic pathway to the pyrrolinones 24 and 25.

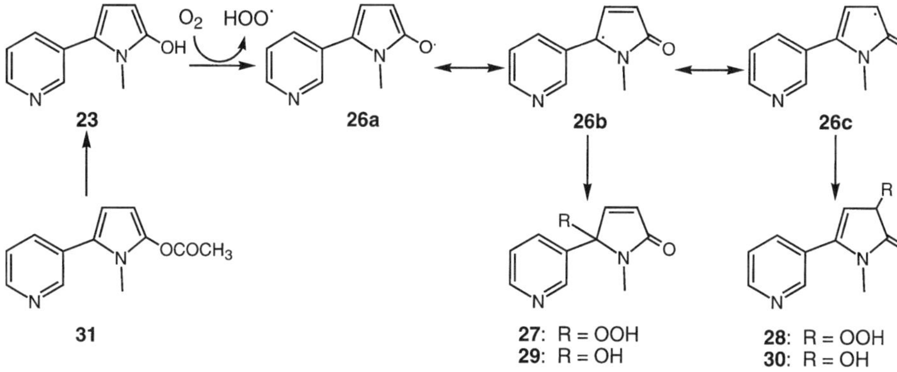

Figure 6-7. Postulated autoxidation pathway for β-nicotyrine metabolite **23**.

an electron and proton (hydrogen atom equivalent) from the hydroxypyrrole tautomer **23** to O_2 leads to the resonance stabilized radical **26a** ↔ **26b** ↔ **26c** and the superoxide radical anion (O_2·⁻) or its conjugate acid, the hydroperoxy radical (HOO·). Radical recombination gives hydroperoxides **27** and **28,** which can undergo hydrolysis to the hydroxypyrrolinones **29** and **30**. The participation of radical intermediates in this chemistry was well documented by studies in which the stable acetoxypyrrole derivative **31** was shown to undergo hydrolysis to **23** and, hence, the pyrrolinones **24** and **25,** which in the presence of O_2, gave the 5-hydroxy-3-pyrrolinone **29**. When this chemistry was examined in the presence of a radical trapping agent, strong electron spin resonance signals were observed that could be assigned to an adduct between the radical trap and a carbon-centered radical derived from **31**. The possible metabolic formation of β-nicotyrine from (S)-nicotine in aldehyde oxidase–deficient lung tissue, and the subsequent generation of radical intermediates from the autoxidation of β-nicotyrine metabolites, suggest that this biotransformation sequence could account for, at least in part, the observed binding of radiolabeled (S)-nicotine to microsomal proteins.

Researchers then focused attention on the in vivo metabolic fate of β-nicotyrine. HPLC analysis of the urine obtained from a treated rabbit showed several minor peaks and one major peak. This principal metabolite displayed HPLC–diode array and GC-EI mass spectral characteristics, indistinguishable from those of *trans*-3-hydroxycotinine **(18),** that is, the principal urinary metabolite of (S)-nicotine. Thorough structural analyses, however, provided an opportunity for researchers to document that the urinary metabolite of β-nicotyrine is the diastereoisomeric species *cis*-3-hydroxycotinine **(33)** (Fig. 6-8). Thus, the pyrrolinones **24** and **25** are probably intermediates in this biotransformation because administration of the acetoxy-β-nicotyrine derivative **31** (the latent form of the pyrrolinones) led to the excretion of large quantities of the *cis*-3-hydroxycotinine metabolite. In addition, smaller amounts of the isomeric 5-hydroxycotinine (**34**) were identified in the urine samples of both the β-nicotyrine–treated animals and the acetoxy-β-nicotyrine–treated animals. Consequently, **34** is probably derived from the pyrrolinones **24** and **25**. Researchers suspect that compound **33** arises from the putative 3-hydroxy-4-pyrrolinone species **30,** or the isomeric 3-hydroxy-3-pyrrolinone **32,** via the action of a reductase, possibly of bacterial origins (Fig. 6-8). Supporting evidence for this proposal is the observed excretion of 5-hydroxycotinine (**34**) as a major metabolite by rodents treated with the 5-hydroxy-3-pyrrolinone **29.**

Conclusions

The results of these studies provide evidence for the metabolic transformation of (S)-nicotine to reactive intermediates that could, through structural modification of biomacromolecules, contribute to some of the degenerative processes leading to the adverse health outcomes observed in chronic users of tobacco products. There is particular interest in the possible participation of β-nicotyrine in the metabolic profile of (S)-nicotine, and speculation that long-term exposure to this metabolically unstable pyrrolic compound may be of toxicological interest. Because *cis*-3-hydroxycotinine is derived from β-nicotyrine, and *trans*-3-hydroxycotinine from (S)-cotinine, it may be possible to assess the extent to which humans are exposed to β-nicotyrine by measuring the *cis*-to-*trans* ratio of these two metabolites in the urine of smokers. It also may be of interest to examine the consequences of inhibiting aldehyde oxidase on the metabolic fate of (S)-nicotine in

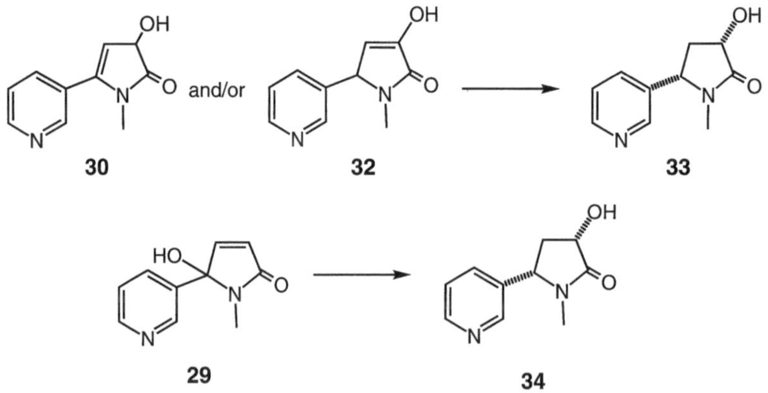

Figure 6-8. Postulated metabolic pathway leading to *cis*-3-hydroxycotinine (**33**).

rodents with particular attention to the potential for enhanced β-nicotyrine formation from (S)-nicotine.

References

1. Ortiz de Montellano PR (ed): *Cytochrome P-450, Structure, Mechanism, and Biochemistry.* New York: Plenum Press, 1986.
2. Dinnocenzo JP, Karki SB, Jones JP: On isotope effects for the cytochrome P-450 oxidation of substituted *N,N,*-dimethylanalines. *Journal of the American Chemical Society* 1993, 115:7113–7116.
3. Guengerich FP, MacDonald TL: Chemical mechanisms of catalysis by cytochrome P-450: A unified view. *Accounts of Chemical Research* 1984, 17:9–16.
4. Beedham C: Molybdenum hydroxylases as drug-metabolizing enzymes. *Drug Metabolism Reviews* 1985, 16:119–156.
5. Murphy PJ: Enzymatic oxidation of nicotine to nicotine $\Delta^{1',5'}$ iminium ion. *Journal of Biological Chemistry.* 1972, 218:2796–2800.
6. Jacob P III, Benowitz NL, Shulgin AT: Recent studies of nicotine metabolism in humans. *Pharmacology, Biochemistry, and Behavior* 1988, 30:249–53.
7. Benowitz NL, Jacob P III: Nicotine metabolism in humans. *Clinical Pharmacology and Therapeutics* 1991, 50:462–464.
8. Lindquist NG, Ullberg S: Autoradiography of intravenously injected ^{14}C-nicotine indicates long-term retention in the respiratory tract. *Nature* 1974, 248:600–601.
9. Waddell W, Marlowe C: Localization of nicotine-^{14}C, cotinine-^{14}C and nicotine-1-oxide in tissues of the mouse. *Drug Metabolism and Disposition* 1976, 4:530–539.
10. Shigenaga MK: *Studies on the Metabolism and Bioactivation of (S)-Nicotine and β-Nicotyrine.* Ph.D. Thesis, University of California, San Francisco, 1991.
11. Shigenaga MK, Jacob P III, Trevor A, Castagnoli N Jr., Benowitz N: Synthesis of specifically labeled (S)-nicotine-5-^{3}H and (S)-cotinine-5-^{3}H by carrier free tritiolysis of the corresponding 5-bromo derivatives. *Journal of Laboratory and Comparative Radiopharmacology* 1987, 24:713–723.
12. Shigenaga MK, Trevor AJ, Castagnoli N Jr: Metabolism-dependent covalent binding of (S)-[5-^{3}H]nicotine to liver and lung microsomal macromolecules. *Drug Metabolism and Disposition* 1988, 16:397–402.
13. Ward DP, Trevor AJ, Adams JD, Baille TC, Castagnoli N, Jr.: Metabolism of phencyclidine. The role of iminium ion formation in covalent binding of rabbit microsomal protein. *Drug Metabolism and Disposition* 1982, 10:690–695.
14. Youngster SK, Sonsalla PK, Sieberg BA, Heikkila RE: Structure–activity of the mechanism of 1-methyl-4-phenyl-1,2,3,6-tetrahydropyridine (MPTP)—Neurotoxicity. I. Evaluation of the biological activity of MPTP analogs. *Journal of Pharmacology and Experimental Therapeutics* 1989, 249:820–828.
15. Kalgutkar AS, Castagnoli K, Hall A, Castagnoli N Jr.: Novel 4-(aryloxy)tetrahydropyridine analogs of MPTP as monoamine oxidase A & B substrates. *Journal of Medicinal Chemistry* 1994, 37:944–949.
16. Liu X: *In Vitro and In Vivo Studies on the Biotransformation of Beta-Nicotyrine, a Minor Tobacco Alkaloid.* Ph.D. Thesis, Virginia Tech, Blacksburg, 1995.
17. Shigenaga MK, Kim BH, Caldera-Munoz P, Cairns T, Jacob P III, Trevor AJ, Castagnoli N Jr.: Liver and lung microsomal metabolism of the tobacco alkaloid β-nicotyrine. *Chemical Research in Toxicology* 1989, 2:282–287.

Chapter 7

Tobacco-Specific Nitrosamines

STEPHEN S. HECHT, ANNA BORUKHOVA,
and STEVEN G. CARMELLA

In 1956, Magee and Barnes[1] described the hepatocarcinogenicity of dimethylnitrosamine, providing the first example of nitrosamine carcinogenesis. Since that landmark study, the broad-ranging and potent carcinogenic activities of more than 200 nitrosamines in at least 40 animal species have been firmly established, and there is substantial evidence that nitrosamines are also responsible for a large number of human cancers.[2–7]

Nitrosamines form readily by nitrosation of secondary and tertiary amines. Such reactions occur in tobacco products containing nicotine and related secondary amines such as nornicotine, anabasine, and anatabine. Nicotine nitrosates to produce N'-nitrosonornicotine (NNN), a constituent of cigarette smoke.[8] The nitrosation of nicotine also produces two other primary nitrosamine products, 4-(methylnitrosamino)-1-(3-pyridyl)-1-butanone (NNK) and 4-(methylnitrosamino)-4-(3-pyridyl)-butanal (NNA).[9] NNK and its metabolic reduction product 4-(methylnitrosamino)-1-(3-pyridyl)-1-butanol (NNAL), as well as the reduction and oxidation products of NNA, 4-(methylnitrosamino)-4-(3-pyridyl)-1-butanol (iso-NNAL) and 4-(methylnitrosamino)-4-(3-pyridyl)butyric acid (iso-NNAC), have been detected in tobacco products.[10–12] These nicotine-derived nitrosamines occur in tobacco products together with N'-nitrosoanabasine (NAB) and N'-nitrosoanatabine (NAT).[10–12] Collectively, these are called *tobacco-specific nitrosamines.* Their structures and those of their alkaloid precursors are shown in Figure 7-1.

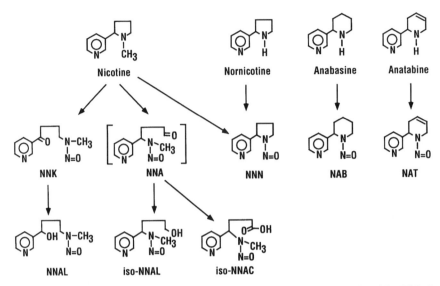

Figure 7-1. Formation of tobacco-specific nitrosamines from tobacco alkaloids. With the exception of NNA, all have been detected in tobacco products.[10–12]

The most prevalent of the tobacco-specific nitrosamines in tobacco products are NNN, NNK, and NAT.[10–12] These compounds occur in substantial quantities in both unburned tobacco and tobacco smoke. Smaller amounts of NNAL, iso-NNAL, iso-NNAC, and NAB are also present in certain tobacco products. Carcinogenicity studies have demonstrated that NNK and its metabolic reduction product NNAL are the most active compounds of this group.[10–12] NNK and NNAL are potent pulmonary carcinogens, inducing adenocarcinoma in rats and mice independent of route of administration. Dose–response studies with NNK have shown that its ability to induce lung tumors extends to total doses as low as 1.8 mg/kg in the rat, a value not dissimilar to that of the exposure of a smoker to NNK.[13,14] NNK is also a strong pulmonary and transplacental carcinogen in the Syrian golden hamster. Secondary target tissues of NNK include nasal cavity, liver, and pancreas in the rat. NNN also possesses considerable carcinogenic activity, inducing tumors of the esophagus in the rat when administered in drinking water and tumors of the nasal cavity when given by subcutaneous injection. NNN causes lung adenomas in mice, tumors of the trachea and nasal cavity in Syrian golden hamsters, and nasal cavity tumors in minks. A mixture of NNK and NNN applied by oral swabbing in the rat induces oral cavity and lung tumors. NAB is also an esophageal carcinogen in the rat, but its activity is less than that of NNN. No strong evidence of carcinogenic activity has been documented for iso-NNAL, iso-NNAC, or NAT.

The carcinogenic properties of tobacco-specific nitrosamines have recently been reviewed.[12] The data strongly support the conclusion that tobacco-specific nitrosamines are among the principal causative factors for cancers of the lung, oral cavity, esophagus, and pancreas associated with tobacco use.[6] The possibility that tobacco-specific nitrosamines could be formed in vivo upon exposure to nicotine is considered in this chapter.

Endogenous nitrosation of nicotine: Previous studies

The formation of nitrosamines occurs readily in laboratory animals upon administration of nitrite and secondary amines.[15] Human exposure to nitrite occurs through the diet, via reduction of dietary nitrate and from endogenously produced nitric oxide.[16,17]

Extensive studies have demonstrated that nitrosamine formation occurs in humans.[18] Thus, nitrosoproline and related sulfur-containing nitrosamino acids can be quantified in human urine. Their levels increase upon ingestion of nitrate and proline and are attenuated by nitrosation inhibitors such as ascorbic acid. Endogenous formation of nitrosoproline has been associated with a number of exposure scenarios linked to cancer risk, including cigarette smoking. It has been suggested that tobacco-specific nitrosamines could be formed endogenously from nicotine, but no data support this hypothesis.[10–12]

Nicotine can be nitrosated under mild conditions to produce NNK, NNN, and NNA.[9] However, the yields are low, and the rate of nitrosation is markedly slower than that of nornicotine or anabasine.[19,20] Nitrosation of nicotine was not observed in simulated saliva or gastric juice.[21] One of the products of endogenous nicotine nitrosation could be iso-NNAC, formed by metabolism of NNA. This nitrosamine could also form by nitrosation of cotinine.[22] Because iso-NNAC is excreted largely unchanged in the urine and feces of rats, it is a potential monitor of endogenous nitrosation of nicotine.[22,23] However, in a study with smokers and abstinent smokers who ingested nicotine or cotinine, with or without nitrate supplementation, there was no conclusive evidence that endogenous nitrosation had occurred.[23]

Evidence for endogenous nitrosation of nicotine and secondary alkaloids in rats

One way to search for endogenous nitrosation of nicotine is to analyze for metabolites of NNK, NNN, or NNA. Previous studies have shown that NNK is metabolized to NNAL and its glucuronide NNAL-Gluc in rats.[24] NNAL and NNAL-Gluc are excreted in urine. The American Health Foundation researchers developed a sensitive method to quantify NNAL and NNAL-Gluc in human urine, and this method appeared to have the requisite characteristics to test the hypothesis that NNK could be formed endogenously in rats treated with nicotine and nitrite.[14] The protocol for this experiment is summarized in Table 7-1.

Table 7-1. Protocol for investigating the endogenous nitrosation of nicotine in rats

Group	No. of Rats	Treatment
1	5	Nicotine (60 μmol/kg) in pH 3 citrate buffer* NaNO$_2$ (180 μmol/kg) in H$_2$O*
2	3	Nicotine (60 μmol/kg) in pH 3 citrate buffer*
3	3	NaNO$_2$ (180 μmol/kg) in H$_2$O*
4	3	NNK (12 nmol/kg) in pH 3 citrate buffer*

*Twice daily, 4 days (i.g.).

Analysis of urine involves a series of solvent-partitioning and HPLC enrichment steps. The appropriate high performance liquid chromatography (HPLC) fractions are silylated and analyzed by gas chromatography (GC) with a nitrosamine-selective thermal energy analyzer (TEA) detector. Typical results of these analyses are presented in Figure 7-2. NNAL (as its trimethylsilyl (TMS) ether) was readily detected in the urine of the NNK-treated rats, as shown in Figure 7-2A.

In the nicotine-treated rats, peaks corresponding to the injection standard nitrosoguvacoline (NG) and the silylation standard iso-NNAL were observed along with a small peak corresponding to NNAL. The NNAL peak could be explained by the amount of ^{3}H-NNAL added as the internal standard. Thus, no evidence was found to support the idea of NNK formation in the nicotine-treated rats. Similarly, in the rats treated with nicotine plus NaNO$_2$, the peak corresponding to NNAL was accounted for by the internal standard. Thus, no evidence for endoge-

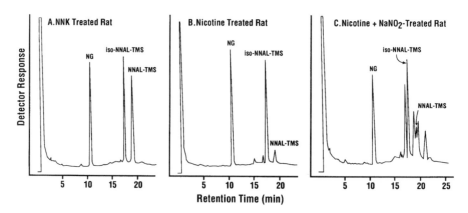

Figure 7-2. Gas chromatography-thermal energy analyzer (GC-TEA) traces obtained upon analysis of urine from rats treated with (A) NNK, (B) nicotine, and (C) nicotine plus NaNo$_2$. NG is nitrosoguvacoline, an injection standard; iso-NNAL-TMS is trimethylsilyl ether of iso-NNAL, a silylation standard; NNal-NNal-TMS is trimethylsilyl ether of NNAL. See text for further details.

nous formation of NNK from nicotine and $NaNO_2$ was shown in this experiment, with a detection limit of approximately $0.4 \times 10^{-4}\%$ nitrosation (based on conversion to NNAL). However, several new peaks were observed in the chromatogram shown in Figure 7-3C. These have not been identified, but may be nitrosamines.

Other HPLC fractions from the urine of the rats treated with nicotine and $NaNO_2$ were also analyzed by GC-TEA. In two fractions, peaks corresponding in retention time to NNN (Fig. 7-3A) as well as NAT and NAB (Fig. 7-3B) were observed. The identities of these peaks have been confirmed by comparisons of their GC retention times to those of standards using both packed and capillary columns, by their HPLC retention times, and by GC–mass spectrometry (MS) with selected ion monitoring. These compounds were not observed in the urine of the rats treated with nicotine or $NaNO_2$ only.

While the formation of NNN in these experiments was plausible as a result of nicotine nitrosation, the presence of NAT and NAB was more difficult to rationalize. Analysis of the nicotine used in the protocol outlined in Figure 7-2 provided an explanation. Although the nicotine was 99.2% pure, it contained small amounts of nornicotine (0.04%), anabasine (0.07%), and anatabine (0.19%). Therefore, the experiment was repeated.

Two groups of three rats each were treated with nicotine and $NaNO_2$. In one group, 99.2% pure nicotine was used, while in the other group synthetic nicotine, not containing detectable nornicotine, anabasine, or anatabine, was used. The results of this experiment are summarized in Table 7-2.

As in the first experiment, NNN, NAB, and NAT were observed in the group treated with the 99.2% pure nicotine and $NaNO_2$. NAB and NAT were not de-

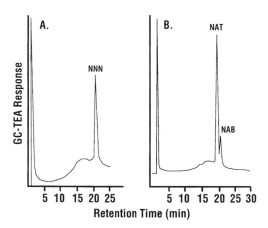

Figure 7-3. GC-TEA traces obtained upon analysis of urine fromn rats treated with nicotine plus $NaNO_2$. The traces in A and B were obtained from HPLC fractions corresponding in retention time to NNN or NAT and NAB, respectively.

tected in the group treated with synthetic nicotine and $NaNO_2$, but NNN was present. Since the nicotine used in this experiment did not contain detectable amounts of nornicotine, it is reasonable to conclude that the NNN detected in the urine of these rats was formed from nicotine. In view of the fact that nicotine can be converted to nornicotine metabolically in rats,[25] it seems likely that NNN was formed by endogenous nitrosation of metabolically produced nornicotine.

The yields of the nitrosamines are summarized in Table 7-2. Previous studies have shown that doses of NNN ranging from 3 to 300 mg/kg are extensively metabolized in rats, with only 3%–5% of the unchanged NNN being excreted in the urine.[26] Therefore, the amount of NNN actually formed by endogenous nitrosation is at least 20 times higher than the amount found in urine. Similar considerations likely apply to NAB and NAT, although their metabolic fates in rats have not been extensively documented.[27] The yield of NNN from nicotine was substantially lower than the yields of NAB and NAT from anabasine and anatabine, which is consistent with expectations. NAB and NAT are secondary amines that would be readily nitrosated.[20] Formation of NNN most likely requires metabolic conversion of nicotine to nornicotine. In rats, approximately 9% of the dose of nicotine is excreted in the urine as nornicotine.[25]

Implications for nicotine safety

The results demonstrate that NNN can be formed in rats treated with nicotine and $NaNO_2$. Moreover, secondary amines present even as minor impurities can be nitrosated. In view of these results, GC and GC-MS were used to analyze the four leading nicotine transdermal systems for anabasine, anatabine, and nornicotine.[28]

Table 7-2. Nitrosamines in urine of two groups of rats, both treated with nicotine and $NaNO_2$

Total Dose/Rat			Nitrosamines in Urine	
Substance	Quantity, mg		Type	Quantity, ng (% yield)
Nicotine (99.2%)				
Nicotine	19.4		NNN	113 (0.53 $\times$ 10^{-3})
Nornicotine	7.8	$\times$ 10^{-3}		
Anabasine	13.6	$\times$ 10^{-3}	NAB	92 (0.68)
Anatabine	37	$\times$ 10^{-3}	NAT	774 (2.1)
Synthetic Nicotine (100%)				
Nicotine	19.4		NNN	100 (0.47 $\times$ 10^{-3})
Nornicotine	0			
Anabasine	0		ND	
Anatabine	0		ND	

One product contained anatabine (0.009% of the amount of nicotine); its presence was confirmed by GC-MS. This product also contained a peak with the same retention time as nornicotine (0.003%). Levels of anabasine, anatabine, and nornicotine in the other products appeared to be less than 0.003% of nicotine, but further quantitation is necessary. Therefore, the formation of NAB, NAT, and NNN from the corresponding secondary amines by endogenous nitrosation does not appear to be a significant problem if the levels of these secondary amines remain low.

However, the potential for nitrosation of nicotine to NNN exists. Nicotine concentrates in the salvia of subjects using the nicotine patch.[29]. Nicotine is metabolized in humans, as in rats, to nornicotine, and it is likely that nornicotine will also be concentrated in saliva.[30] Nitrite is also known to occur in human saliva, with a total exposure of approximately 3 mg/day, excluding endogenous sources.[16] Saliva is swallowed and the stomach provides a favorable pH for nitrosation. Nicotine and nornicotine are ionized and poorly absorbed from the stomach.[31] Therefore, conditions for nitrosation of metabolically formed nornicotine could be favorable in nicotine patch users. It is important to analyze human urine for NNN and its metabolites and to determine whether endogenous nitrosation is a quantitatively significant problem in these individuals.

Conclusions

Tobacco-specific nitrosamines, which are formed from nicotine and other tobacco alkaloids, are present in tobacco products and are likely causative agents for cancers of the lung, oral cavity, esophagus, and pancreas in people who use these produces. NNK, NNN, and NNAL are the most carcinogenic tobacco-specific nitrosamines. The formation of tobacco-specific nitrosamines was examined in rats treated with nicotine and sodium nitrite. The results indicate that NNK and its metabolic reduction product NNAL were not produced under these conditions. However, NNN was detected in the urine of rats treated with nicotine and sodium nitrite. Moreover, trace amounts of anabasine and anatabine, present in the nicotine, were readily nitrosated in these rats. The results demonstrate that nicotine can undergo endogenous nitrosation to produce NNN, probably by way of metabolically produced nicotine, and that secondary amine impurities in nicotine can also be readily nitrosated. Further studies are required to determine whether similar nitrosation reactions occur in people using nicotine replacement products.

Acknowledgments

These studies were supported by grants CA-29580 and CA-44377 from the National Institutes of Health, National Cancer Institute. Special thanks are given to Dhimant Desai and Shantu Amin, American Health Foundation, Organic Synthesis Facility, for providing synthetic nicotine.

References

1. Magee PN, Barnes JM: The production of malignant primary hepatic tumors in the rat by feeding dimethylnitrosamine. *British Journal of Cancer* 1956, 10:114–122.
2. Druckrey H, et al.: Organotrope carcinogen wirkungen bei 65 verschiedenen *N*-nitrosoverbindungen an BD-ratten. *Zeitschrift Krebsforschung* 1967, 69:103–201.
3. Preussmann R, Stewart BW: *N*-nitroso carcinogens. In Searle CE (ed): *Chemical Carcinogens,* 2nd ed, vol 2. Washington, DC: American Chemical Society, 1984, pp 643–828.
4. Lijinsky W: *Chemistry and Biology of N-Nitroso Compounds.* Cambridge: Cambridge University Press, 1992, pp 251–403.
5. Magee PN: The experimental basis for the role of nitroso compounds in human cancer. *Cancer Surveys* 1989, 8:207–239.
6. Hecht SS, Hoffmann D: The relevance of tobacco-specific nitrosamines to human cancer. *Cancer Surveys* 1989, 8:273–294.
7. Reed PI: *N*-nitroso compounds, their relevance to human cancer and further prospects for prevention. *European Journal of Cancer Prevention* 1996, 5(suppl 1):137–147.
8. Hoffmann D, et al.: On the isolation and identification of volatile and non-volatile *N*-nitrosamines and hydrazines in cigarette smoke. In *N-Nitroso Compounds in the Environment,* vol 9. Lyon: IARC Scientific Publications, International Agency for Research on Cancer. 1979, pp 159–165.
9. Hecht SS, et al.: Reaction of nicotine and sodium nitrite: Formation of nitrosamines and fragmentation of the pyrrolidine ring. *Journal of Organic Chemistry* 1978, 43: 72–76.
10. Hoffmann D, Hecht SS: Nicotine-derived *N*-nitrosamines and tobacco related cancer: Current status and future directions. *Cancer Research* 1985, 45:935–944.
11. Hecht SS, Hoffmann D: Tobacco-specific nitrosamines, an important group of carcinogens in tobacco and tobacco smoke. *Carcinogenesis* 1988, 9:875–884.
12. Hoffmann D, et al.: Tobacco-specific *N*-nitrosamines and *areca*-derived *N*-nitrosamines: Chemistry, biochemistry, carcinogenicity, and relevance to humans. *Journal of Toxicology and Environmental Health* 1994, 41:1–52.
13. Belinsky SA, et al.: Dose–response relationship between O^6-methylguanine formation in Clara cells and induction of pulmonary neoplasia in the rat by 4-(methylnitrosamino)-1-(3-pyridyl)-1-butanone. *Cancer Research* 1990, 50:3772–3780.
14. Carmella SG, et al.: Metabolites of the tobacco-specific nitrosamine 4-(methylnitrosamino)-1-(3-pyridyl)-1-butanone in smokers' urine. *Cancer Research* 1993, 53: 721–724.
15. Mirvish SS: Formation of *N*-nitroso compounds: Chemistry, kinetics, and in vivo occurrence. *Toxicology and Applied Pharmacology* 1975, 31:325–351.
16. Assembly of Life Sciences: *The Health Effects of Nitrate, Nitrite, and N-Nitroso Compounds.* Washington, DC: National Academy Press, 1988.
17. Marletta MA: Mammalian synthesis of nitrite, nitrate, nitric oxide, and *N*-nitrosating agents. *Chemical Research in Toxicology* 1988, 1:249–257.
18. Bartsch H, et al.: Human exposure to endogenous *N*-nitroso compounds: Quantitative estimates in subjects at high risk for cancer of the oral cavity, oesophagus, stomach and urinary bladder. *Cancer Surveys* 1989, 8:335–362.
19. Caldwell WS, et al.: The nitrosation of nicotine: A kinetic study. *Chemical Research in Toxicology* 1991, 4:513–516.
20. Mirvish SS, et al.: Kinetics of nornicotine and anabasine nitrosation in relation to N'-

nitrosonornicotine occurrence in tobacco and to tobacco-induced cancer. *Journal of the National Cancer Institute* 1977, 59:1211–1213.

21. Tricker AR, et al.: The occurrence of tobacco-specific nitrosamines in oral tobacco products and their potential formation under simulated gastric conditions. *Food and Chemical Toxicology* 1988, 26:861–865.

22. Djordjevic MV, et al.: Formation of 4-(methylnitrosamino)-4-(3-pyridyl)butyric acid in vitro and in mainstream cigarette smoke. *Journal of Agriculture and Food Chemistry* 1991, 39:209–213.

23. Tricker AR, et al.: Evaluation of 4-(*N*-methylnitrosamino)-4-(3-pyridyl)butyric acid as a potential monitor of endogenous nitrosation of nicotine and its metabolites. *Carcinogenesis* 1993, 14:1409–1414.

24. Morse MA, et al.: Characterization of a glucuronide metabolite of 4-(methylnitrosamino)-1-(3-pyridyl)-1-butanone (NNK) and its dose-dependent excretion in the urine of mice and rats. *Carcinogenesis* 1990, 11:1819–1823.

25. Kyerematen GA, et al.: Radiometric high performance liquid chromatographic assay for nicotine and twelve of its metabolites. *Journal of Chromatography* 1987, 419: 191–203.

26. Hecht SS, et al.: Comprehensive analysis of urinary metabolites of *N'*-nitrosonornicotine. *Carcinogenesis* 1981, 2:833–838.

27. Hecht SS, Young R: Regiospecificity in the metabolism of the homologous cyclic nitrosamines, *N'*-nitrosonornicotine and *N'*-nitrosoanabasine. *Carcinogenesis* 1982, 3:1195–1199.

28. Gora ML: Nicotine transdermal systems. *Annals of Pharmacotherapy* 1993, 27: 742–749.

29. Rose JE, et al.: Saliva nicotine as an index of plasma levels in nicotine patch users. *Therapeutic Drug Monitoring* 1993, 15:431–435.

30. Benowitz NL, et al.: Nicotine metabolic profile in man: Comparison of cigarette smoking and transdermal nicotine. *Journal of Pharmacology and Experimental Therapeutics* 1994, 268:296–303.

31. U.S. Surgeon General: *The Health Consequences of Smoking: Nicotine Addiction.* Washington, DC: U.S. Department of Health and Human Services, U.S. Government Printing Office, 1988.

Chapter 8

Nicotine and Lung Cancer

HILDEGARD M. SCHULLER

Lung cancer is the most common malignancy in both men and women and demonstrates a strong association with smoking.[1,2] A large number of chemicals that cause lung cancer in experimental animals have been identified in cigarette smoke.[2] Extensive research into the mechanisms of action of these chemical carcinogens has shown that their reactive metabolites interact with DNA to form DNA adducts.[3,4] Among these, O^6-methylguanine is a prominent adduct formed from 4-(methylnitrosamino)-1-(3-pyridyl)-1-butanone (NNK)[4], the most potent and abundant carcinogen contained in tobacco products. The formation of this particular adduct has been implicated in the activation of the Ki-*ras* protoonco-gene.[5] This member of the *ras* gene family is most frequently mutated in human[6] and experimentally induced[5,7] non-small cell lung cancer (NSCLC), an event considered a critical mediator in the genesis of this cancer type.[5,8]

However, the mechanisms of lung carcinogenesis are far from understood. One major question is if the dose levels of NNK required for tumor induction in animals (1–20 mg/kg body weight) and the detection of promutagenic adducts in tissues and cells (concentrations in the 5–100 µM range) are, in fact, reached in lung cells of smokers when the mainstream smoke concentration of NNK is only between 5 and 97 ng per cigarette.[9] Moreover, small cell lung cancer (SCLC), a histological tumor type that is almost exclusively found in smokers,[1] lacks point mutations in the *ras* gene and demonstrates overexpression/amplification of *myc* family genes instead.[10] None of the chemicals contained in cigarette smoke induce molecular changes in this gene family experimentally, and the genesis of SCLC is the least well understood among all lung cancers.

Chronic non-neoplastic lung disease is a risk factor for the development of lung cancer.[11] This disease complex includes chronic bronchitis and bronchiolitis, chronic obstructive pulmonary disease, and emphysema. Such diseases typically impair the pulmonary ventilation, resulting in elevated concentrations of CO_2 at the expense of O_2. Pulmonary neuroendocrine (PNE) cells have been shown to respond via an oxygen receptor-mediated mechanism with the secretion of the biogenic amine 5-hydroxytryptamine (5-HT, serotonin) and the neuropeptide mammalian bombesin (MB) in vivo and in vitro upon exposure to reduced O_2 concentration or increase in CO_2 (12–14). As both of these products are autocrine growth factors for PNE cells,[15,16] this enhanced secretory activity is always accompanied by an increase in PNE cell proliferation. In addition, MB is also a growth factor for non-neuroendocrine epithelial lung cells.[17] Chronic stimulation of O_2 receptor-initiated growth factor secretion by PNE cells may thus contribute to the observed high overall lung cancer risk in individuals with chronic lung disease.

The "signal transduction model of carcinogenesis" implies that, in addition to the widely studied abnormalities at the gene levels malfunctioning, signal transduction components upstream, such as second messengers and receptors, may play a crucial role in the genesis of cancer.[18]. In light of epidemiological and experimental evidence for an involvement of O_2 receptor-mediated signal transduction pathways in the genesis of lung cancer, the potential interaction of tobacco-associated chemicals with such regulatory pathways in normal and neoplastic PNE cells has been addressed. Accordingly, hamsters with impaired pulmonary ventilation due to hyperoxic lung injury (emphysema, fibrosis) were shown to develop lung tumors with a neuroendocrine phenotype when treated with N-nitroso-diethylamine (DEN)[19,20] or NNK,[21] while healthy animals developed Clara cell–derived adenomas and adenocarcinmas upon exposure to identical nitrosamine treatments. Subsequently, DEN and NNK have been shown to compete successfully with nicotine for nicotinic-binding sites in receptor-binding assays with cell membrane fractions from hamster lung homogenates.[22] These findings suggest that the simultaneous stimulation of signal transduction pathways, initiated by nicotinic acetylcholine receptors (nAChRs) and O_2 receptors, may be important events for the initiation and progression of neuroendocrine lung tumors.

As nicotine is a classic agonist of the nAChR, most of the experiments to test this working hypothesis included comparisons between the effects of NNK and nicotine. A few laboratories, at the same time, began focusing their attention on the potential impact of nicotine on pulmonary carcinogenesis. The data emerging from these experiments suggest that, in addition to its well-documented effects on the cardiovascular and central nervous systems, nicotine may modulate tobacco-associated lung carcinogenesis.

Potential tumor-promoting effects of nicotine

The parasympathetic branch of the autonomic nervous system regulates the secretion of calcitonin by PNE cells in vivo via stimulation of nicotinic receptors by the neurotransmitter acetylcholine.[23] As this effect was accompanied by hyperplasia of PNE cells, although calcitonin is not a growth factor for these cells,[24] we assumed that the secretion of one or several autocrine growth factors was also activated by a nicotinic cholinergic pathway. In support of this hypothesis, in vitro studies with fetal hamster PNE cells, and several cell lines derived from human neuroendocrine lung cancers, demonstrated an increase in cell number and ^{3}H-thymidine incorporation in response to nicotine and NNK, which was inhibited by antagonists of receptors for MB and 5-HT.[25] These findings indicate that both of these autocrine growth factors are secreted by normal and neoplastic PNE cells in response to nicotinic receptor stimulation.

This interpretation was corroborated by two laboratories reporting a significant stimulation of SCLC cell proliferation in response to nicotine, accompanied by an increase in 5-HT levels in the culture media.[26,27] However, one laboratory reported no direct effect of nicotine on cell proliferation but observed a reversal of opioid-induced inhibition of SCLC cell proliferation by nicotine.[28] Subsequently, the investigators involved have identified the molecular mechanism responsible for this effect as an inhibition of opioid-induced apoptosis by nicotine.[29] Stimulation of cell proliferation and inhibition of programmed cell death increase the number of viable cells. Accordingly, all of these data suggest a tumor-promoting effect of nicotine on SCLC.

It seemed odd that three independent laboratories consistently observed a proliferative response of normal and neoplastic PNE cells to nicotine, while one other laboratory consistently failed to see this effect. Detailed discussions with all investigators soon revealed that all laboratories that had observed a proliferative response to nicotine routinely maintained their PNE cells at relatively high CO_2 concentrations (8%–10%),[25–27] while the unsuccessful group routinely used a culture environment of 5% CO_2.[28] The intra-alveolar concentration of CO_2 in healthy adult individuals is 5%, while it is significantly higher (8%–30%, depending on the severity of the condition) in individuals with chronic lung disease.[30]

Cellular responses observed in the experiments conducted in the high CO_2 atmosphere can be considered the in vitro correlate of such reactions in individuals with moderately impaired pulmonary ventilation due to chronic lung disease. On the other hand, experimental designs utilizing an atmosphere of 5% CO_2 are good model systems for the study of cellular reactions in the lungs of healthy individuals.

Further analyses demonstrated a concentration-dependent and saturable proliferative response to CO_2 by normal and neoplastic PNE cells and identified activation of protein kinase C and c-*fos* as downstream events upon stimulation of the

O_2 receptor by 10% CO_2.[25] Antagonists of receptors for 5-HT and MB yielded significant inhibition of the proliferative response to CO_2, thus identifying secretion and re-uptake of these two growth factors as additional mediating factors.[25] Nicotine and NNK both failed to stimulate the proliferation of normal and neoplastic PNE cells in an environment of 5% CO_2, while both agents significantly potentiated the proliferative response of these cells to 10% CO_2.[25] The promoting effects of nicotine and NNK on CO_2-induced cell proliferation were completely inhibited by hexamethonium but not decamethonium, thus identifying the nAChR involved as a neuronal subtype of the nAChR family. Receptor-binding assays with the human SCLC line NCI-H69 demonstrated the expression of a functional neuronal nAChR with the α-bungarotoxin (α-BTX)–sensitive α7-binding domain in these cells.[26,31] Preincubation of cells with α-BTX completely inhibited the proliferative response of this cell line to nicotine and NNK.[31] These findings suggest that nicotine and NNK both stimulate these cells via binding to the α7-nAChR. In support of this hypothesis, NNK competed successfully for nicotinic binding sites against ^{125}I–α-BTX in receptor-binding assays.[12]

These findings are important as they identified, for the first time, a defined subtype of the neuronal nAChR family as the binding site for the tobacco-specific nitrosamine NNK. Competitive nAChR agonists such as acetylcholine and nicotine are internalized and enzymatically degraded following binding to the nAChR.[32,33] It is therefore conceivable that binding of NNK to the α7-nAChR serves as a mechanism for the selective uptake of this carcinogen by cells expressing this receptor type, thus yielding substantially higher intracellular concentrations of the nitrosamine than cells not expressing this receptor.

In light of the fact that well-differentiated neoplastic PNE cells are able to metabolize nitrosamines,[34] substantially higher concentrations of reactive metabolites and DNA adducts could be generated in such cells than would accumulate if an even distribution of NNK by passive diffusion were assumed. However, we have shown that the SCLC lines that respond with cell proliferation in an environment of high CO_2 to NNK are unable to metabolize nitrosamines.[35] Moreover, nicotine, which does not form carcinogenic DNA adducts, yielded a similar or even greater proliferative response in the cell proliferation assays.[25,36] These findings indicate that the nAChR-mediated proliferative effects of NNK on PNE cells in the presence of a stimulated O_2 receptor are mediated by the parent nitrosamine and do not require metabolic activation. However, a stimulation of cell proliferation does not necessarily imply carcinogenic potency. Accordingly, identification of nAChR-initiated cell proliferation as a promoting factor in the genesis of lung cancer would require the experimental induction of lung cancer with a nicotinic agonist that does not form carcinogenic DNA adducts in an animal model of chronic non-neoplastic lung disease.

An experiment was conducted in which hamsters with experimentally induced hyperoxic lung injury were treated with multiple subcutaneous injections of nicotine at a dose (0.1 mg/kg) that can be achieved in a moderate smoker. A significant number (6 of 20) of these animals developed lung tumors with foci of positive immunoreactivity for 5-HT and neuron-specific enolase, as well as nasal cavity tumors.[37] These data strongly support the hypothesis that chronic stimulation of the nAChR by nicotinic agonists in the diseased lung, rich in CO_2, contributes to the high burden of lung cancer observed in smokers.

The relative contributions of nicotine and NNK to this effect are not clear. Cigarettes contain between 5,000 and 30,000 times more nicotine than NNK.[3,9] The odds are thus very much in favor of nicotine when both agents compete for identical nicotinic-binding sites in a smoker's lung. However, our receptor-binding assays have shown that equimolar or lower concentrations of NNK compete successfully for the $\alpha7$-binding sites with ^{125}I–α-BTX.[31]

The affinity of nicotine to the $\alpha7$-receptor is about 100 times lower than that of α-BTX.[38,39] In addition, the $\alpha7$-receptor represents a small minority, about 10%, of the nAChR family in the central nervous system.[38] Unfortunately, it is unknown at this time which cell types in the lung express this receptor type. It is also not known whether NNK binds to nAChR subtypes other than $\alpha7$. These questions have to be answered to allow assessment of the relative contributions of NNK and nicotine to lung cancer.

Potential tumor-inhibiting effects of nicotine

Long-term exposure to nicotinic agonists can result in desensitization of the nAChR, and there are pronounced interindividual differences in the susceptibilities of smokers to this desensitizing effect.[40] On the other hand, the nAChR-mediated stimulation of PNE cell growth by nicotine and NNK in vitro was observed in short-term experiments with single applications of these tobacco constituents followed by observation periods of up to 10 days.[16,25–27] Similarly, the nAChR-mediated inhibition of induced apoptosis was observed in cells exposed to nicotine for relatively short periods of time.[28,29] The tumor induction experiments in hamsters with hyperoxic lung injury had treatment regimens in which nicotine[37] or the nitrosamines[19–21] were given at intervals of 2–3 days between each injection. All of these experimental designs are unlikely to affect the sensitivity of the nAChR and should be considered model systems for the study of functional aspects of unaltered receptors. It is possible that in individuals whose nAChR has been desensitized by regular nicotine abuse the trophic responses to nicotine and NNK are greatly diminished or even blocked, an effect that could inhibit lung cancer growth.

NNK is the most potent chemical carcinogen contained in tobacco products.[22] With respect to the overabundance of nicotine compared with NNK in cigarettes,[9] the competition of these two agonists for nicotinic-binding sites in a smoker's lung may therefore inhibit the cellular uptake of the nitrosamine. This, in turn, would inhibit the formation of carcinogenic DNA adducts, thus reducing the lung cancer risk. In addition, nicotine and NNK both undergo metabolism by the same oxidative enzyme systems.[22,41] In the presence of an overabundance of nicotine, competition for these enzymes could further reduce the amount of carcinogenic DNA adducts formed from NNK. In support of this interpretation, it has been shown by several laboratories that the simultaneous exposure to nicotine and NNK reduces the amount of reactive metabolites formed from NNK.[22,42]

Conclusions

Lung cancer continues to be the major cause of cancer deaths in industrialized nations. Recent reports strongly suggest that chronic non-neoplastic lung diseases such as bronchitis, bronchiolitis, chronic obstructive pulmonary disease, emphysema, and asthma may be more of a risk factor for lung cancer in smokers than smoking per se.[11] As exemplified by in vitro and in vivo experiments, elevated CO_2 concentrations, as are found in the poorly ventilated diseased lung, are essential to rendering normal and neoplastic PNE cells susceptible to the stimulating effects of nicotine and NNK on growth factor secretion and cell proliferation and to inducing neuroendocrine lung tumors in experimental animals.

Although cigarette smoke contains a host of carcinogens and respiratory tract irritants, only some smokers develop such chronic respiratory tract diseases. Similarly, not every individual exposed to air pollutants believed to be among the etiological factors for this disease complex[43] actually develops the disease. The recent discovery that lung tissue of individuals with chronic non-neoplastic lung disease, as well as lung tumors, demonstrates a decrease in or absence of expression of neutral endopeptidase[12] points to a common risk factor for both disease complexes. The enzyme neutral endopeptidase hydrolyzes all growth factors of the neuropeptide family, including MB. Absence or downregulation of this enzyme causes increased persistence of these growth factors in cells,[12] thus potentiating their mitogenic effects. Although the mechanisms responsible for these altered levels of neutral endopeptidase expression are obscure, there is some evidence that they may be genetically linked.[12]

Studies in laboratory animals have amply demonstrated that chemical carcinogens, such as NNK contained in tobacco products, can cause NSCLC in healthy animals without the promoting effects of chronic non-neoplastic lung disease. However, the high dose levels of carcinogens used in these studies are unlikely to be reached in a smoker's lung. It is likely that in the diseased lung with high CO_2 concentrations, considerably lower carcinogen doses induce this histological cancer type because the growth of non-neuroendocrine lung cells is also stimulated by the joint stimulation of MB secretion via the nAChR and O_2 receptor signaling pathways of PNE cells.

Similarly, the development of lung tumors with a neuroendocrine phenotype is greatly facilitated by stimulation of the 5-HT and MB autocrine loops via the nAChR and O_2 receptor and possibly by selective receptor uptake of NNK as well, resulting in a high yield of carcinogenic DNA adducts. However, it is to be expected that the responses to identical levels of exposure of tobacco products will vary greatly among individuals. Interindividual variations in the sensitivity of the α7-nAChR, as well as the receptors for O_2, 5-HT, and MB, and individual differences in the expression of neutral endopeptidase undoubtedly have a profound effect on the responses of normal and diseased lungs to tobacco products. Both nicotine and NNK have the potential to increase the lung cancer risk, although their relative contributions to the lung cancer burden observed in smokers are far from clear at this time. On the other hand, nicotine may, in some cases, protect against the carcinogenic effects of NNK.

References

1. Weiss W: Epidemiology of lung cancer. In Reznik-Schüller HM (ed): *Comparative Respiratory Tract Carcinogenesis.* Boca Raton: CRC Press, 1983, pp 1–18.
2. Wynder EL, Hoffmann D: Smoking and lung cancer: Scientific challenges and opportunities. *Cancer Research* 1994, 54:5284–5295.
3. Hecht SS, Hoffmann D: Tobacco-specific nitrosamines, an important group of carcinogens in tobacco and tobacco smoke. *Carcinogenesis* 1990, 9:875–884.
4. Hecht SS, Carmella SG, Foiles PG, Murphy SE: Tobacco-specific nitrosamine adducts. *Environmental Health Perspectives* 1993, 99:57–63.
5. Belinsky SA, Devereux TR, Maranpot RR, Stoner GD, Anderson MW: Relationship between the formation of promutagenic adducts and the activation of the Ki-*ras* protooncogene in lung tumors of A/J mice treated with nitrosamines. *Cancer Research* 1989, 49:5305–5311.
6. Mitsudomi T, Viallet J, Mulshine JL, Linnoila RI, Minna JD, Gazdar AF: Mutations of *ras* genes distinguish a subset of non-small cell lung cancer cell lines from small cell lung cancer cell lines. *Oncogene* 1991, 6:1353–1362.
7. Oreffo VIC, Lin HW, Gumerlock PH, Kraegel SA, Witschi HP: Mutational analysis of a dominant oncogene (c-Ki-*ras*-2) and a tumor suppressor gene (*p53*) in hamster lung tumourigenesis. *Molecular Carcinogenesis* 1992, 6:199–202.
8. Rhodenius S, Slebos RJC, Boot AJM, Evers SG, Mooi WJ, Wagenaar SSC, van Bodegom PCh, Bos JL: Incidence and possible clinical significance of K-*ras* oncogene activation in adenocarcinoma of the lung. *Cancer Research* 1988, 48:5738–5741.
9. Fischer S, Castonguay A, Kaiserman M, Spiegelhalder B, Pressmann R: Tobacco-specific nitrosamines in Canadian cigarettes. *Journal of Cancer Research and Clinical Oncology* 1990, 116:563–568.
10. Wong AJ, Ruppert JM, Eggleston J, Hamilton SR, Baylin SB, Vogelstein B: Gene amplification of C-*myc* and N-*myc* in small cell carcinoma of the lung. *Science* 1986, 233:461–464. 11. Weiss W: COPD and lung cancer. In Cherniak NS (ed): *Chronic Obstructive Pulmonary Disease.* Philadelphia: WB Saunders, 1991, pp 344–347.
12. Cutz E, Gillan JE, Track NS: Pulmonary endocrine cells in the developing human lung and during neonatal adaptation. In Becker KL, Gazdar AF (eds): *The Endocrine Lung in Health and Disease.* Philadelphia: WB Saunders. 1984, pp 210–231.

13. Johnson DE, Georgieff MK: Pulmonary perspective: Neuroendocrine cells in health and disease. *American Review of Respiratory Diseases* 1988, 249:825–830.

14. Youngson C, Nurse C, Yeger H, Cutz E: Oxygen sensing in airway chemorecptors. *Nature* 1993, 365:153–155.

15. Gazdar AF: The biology of endocrine lung tumors. In Becker KL, Gazdar AF (eds): *The Endocrine Lung in Health and Disease.* Philadelphia: WB Saunders, 1984, pp 448–459.

16. Schuller HM, Hegedus TJ: Effects of endogenous and tobacco-related amines and nitrosamines on cell growth and morphology of a cell line derived from a human neuroendocrine lung cancer. *Toxicology In Vitro* 1989, 3:37–43.

17. Siegfried JM, Guentert PJ, Gaither AL: Effects of bombesin and gastrin-releasing peptide on human bronchial epithelial cells from a series of donors: Individual variation and modulation by bombesin analogues. *Anatomical Record* 1993, 236:241–247.

18. Schuller HM: The signal transduction model of carcinogenesis. *Biochemical Pharmacology* 1991, 42:1511–1523.

19. Schuller HM, Becker KL, Witschi HP: An animal model for neuroendocrine lung cancer. *Carcinogenesis* 1988, 7:293–296.

20. Schuller HM, Correa E, Orloff M, Reznik GK: Successful chemotherapy of experimental neuroendocrine lung tumors in hamsters with an antagonist of Ca^{2+}/calmodulin. *Cancer Research* 1990, 50:1645–1649.

21. Schuller HM, Witschi HP, Nylen ES, Joshi PA, Correa E, Becker KL: Pathobiology of NNK-induced lung tumors in hamsters and the modulating effect of hyperoxia. *Cancer Research* 1990, 50:1960–1965.

22. Schuller HM, Castonguay A, Orloff M, Rossignol G: Modulation of the uptake and metabolism of 4-(methylnitrosamino)-1-(3-pyridyl)-1-butanone (NNK) by nicotine in hamster lung. *Cancer Research* 1991, 51:2009–2014.

23. Nylen ES, Linnoila IR, Becker KL: Prenatal cholinergic stimulation of pulmonary neuroendocrine cells by nicotine. *Acta Physiologica Scandinavica* 1988, 132: 117–118.

24. Becker KL, Silva OL, Snider RH, Moore CF, Geehoed GW, Nash D, O'Neill WJ, Fink RJ, Murphy TM, Klass EM, Rohatgi PK: The pathophysiology of calcitonin. In Becker KL, Gazdar AF (eds): *The Endocrine Lung in Health and Disease.* Philadelphia: WB Saunders, 1994, pp 277–299.

25. Schuller HM: Carbon dioxide potentiates the mitogenic effects of nicotine and its carcinogenic derivative NNK in normal and neoplastic neuroendocrine lung cells via stimulation of autocrine and protein kinase C–dependent mitogenic pathways. *Neurotoxicology* 1994, 15:877–886.

26. Cattaneo MG, Codignola A, Vicenti LM, Clementi F, Sher E: Nicotine stimulates a serotonergic autocrine loop in human small cell lung carcinoma. *Cancer Research* 1993, 53:5566–5568.

27. Quik M, Chan J, Patrick J: α-Bungarotoxin blocks the nicotinic receptor mediated increase in cell number in a neuroendocrine cell line. *Brain Research* 1994, 655: 161–167.

28. Maneckje R, Minna JD: Opioid and nicotine affect growth regulation of human lung cancer cell lines. *Proceedings of the National Academy of Science* 1990, 87: 3294–3298.

29. Maneckjee R, Minna JD: Opioids induce while nicotine suppresses apoptosis in human lung cancer cells. *Cell Growth and Differentiation* 1994, 5:1033–1040.

30. Lamberstson CJ: The atmosphere and gas exchange with the lungs and blood. In vol.

2. Mountcastle VB (ed): *Medical Physiology.* Saint Louis: CV Mosby, 1974, pp 1372–1398.

31. Schuller HM, Orloff M: Tobacco-Specific Carcinogenic Nitrosamines. Ligands for Nicotinic Acetylcholine Receptors in Human Lung Cancer Cells. *Biochemical Pharmacology* 1998 (in press).

32. Taylor P: Agents acting at the neurohumoral junction and autonomic ganglia. In Gilman AG, Rall TW, Nies AS, Taylor P (eds): *The Pharmacological Basis Of Therapeutics.* New York: Pergamon Press, 1990, pp 187–220.

33. Berg DG, Zhang ZW, Conroy WG, Pugh PC, Corriveau RA, Romano SJ, Rathouz MM, Huang S, Vijayaraghavan S: Quik M, Adlkofer FX, Thurau K (eds): *Expression, function, and Regulation of Neuronal Nicotinic Acetylcholine Receptors Containing the α7 Gene Product.* Basel: Birkhäuser Verlag, 1995, pp 61–70.

34. Hegedus TJ, Falzon M, Margaretten N, Gazdar AF, Schuller HM: Inhibition of *N*-diethylnitrosamine metabolism in human lung cancer cell lines with features of well differentiated pulmonary neuroendocrine cells. *Biochemical Pharmacology* 1987, 36: 3339–3343.

35. Falzon M, McMahon JB, Gazdar AF, Schuller HM: Preferential metabolism of *N*-nitrosodiethylamine by two cell lines derived from human pulmonary adenocarcinomas. *Carcinogenesis* 1986, 7:17–22.

36. Schuller HM: Cell type specific, receptor-mediated modulation of growth kinetics in human lung cancer cell lines by nicotine and tobacco-related nitrosamines. *Biochemical Pharmacology* 1989, 38:3439–3442.

37. Schuller HM, McGavin MD, Orloff M, Riechert A, Porter B: Simultaneous exposure to nicotine and hyperoxia causes tumors in hamsters. *Laboratory Investigation* 1995, 73:448–456.

38. Gotti C, Hanke W, Moretti R, Longhi B, Balestra L, Briscini L, Clementi F: α-Bungarotoxin receptor subtypes. In Quik M, Adlkofer FX, Thurau K (eds): *Effects of Nicotine on Biological Systems.* Basel: Birkhäuser Verlag, 1995, pp 37–44.

39. Lindstrom J, Anand R, Peng X, Gerzanich V: Neuronal nicotinic receptor structure and function. In Quik M, Adlkofer FX, Thurau K (eds): *Effects of Nicotine on Biological Systems.* Basel: Birkhäuser Verlag, 1995, pp 45–52.

40. Rosencrans JA, Karan LD, James JR: Nicotine is a discriminative stimulus: Individual variability to acute tolerance and the role of receptor desensitization. In Clark PBS, Quik M, Adlkofer F, Thurau K (eds): *Effects of Nicotine on Biological Systems.* Basel: Birkhäuser Verlag, 1995, pp 219–224.

41. Benowitz NL, Jacob P III: Metabolism, pharmacokinetics, and pharmacodynamics of nicotine in man. In Van Loon GR, Iwamoto ET, Davis L (eds): *Tobacco Smoke and Nicotine.* New York: Plenum Press, 1987, pp 357–374.

42. Kutzer C, Richter E, Oehlmann C, Atawodi SE: Effect of nicotine and cotinine on NNK metabolism in rats. In Clarke PBS, Quik M, Adlkofer F, Thurau K (eds): *Effects of Nicotine on Biological Systems.* Basel: Birkhäuser Verlag, 1995, pp 385–390.

43. Rusznak C, Devalia JL, Davies R: The impact of air pollution on allergic disease. *Allergy* 1994, 49(suppl 18):S21–S27.

Nicotine
and Reproduction

Cigarette smoking causes reproductive disturbances during pregnancy and after pregnancy, impacting the health of the neonate. Smoking during pregnancy is associated with an increased risk of spontaneous abortion, intrauterine growth retardation, placental abruption, placenta previa, prematurity, and infant death. The risk of sudden infant death syndrome is greater for infants of mothers who smoke, and there is concern about long-lasting impairment of cognitive and other brain functions in the offspring of smokers.

Nicotine is believed to contribute to some reproductive disturbances. In Part III, the mechanisms by which nicotine could contribute to adverse effects are reviewed, the methodology for assessing fetal exposure to nicotine is examined, and the research on the effects of short-term nicotine replacement therapy during pregnancy is discussed. Part III also provides background information for designing future studies of nicotine-based smoking cessation therapies during pregnancy.

Chapter 9

The Impact of Fetal Nicotine Exposure on Nervous System Development and Its Role in Sudden Infant Death Syndrome

THEODORE A. SLOTKIN

The adverse effects of tobacco on the offspring of women smokers have a long history. In addition to fetal and infant mortality, the most notable ones associated with nicotine are increased learning disabilities and attention deficit and hyperactivity disorders—even when birth weight is normal—because nicotine targets the brain.

The availability of alternative forms of nicotine compels exploration of whether pregnant women who smoke should use nicotine replacement medication for smoking cessation. While it is somewhat difficult to extrapolate from animal models to humans, and intake of carbon monoxide and other toxins in cigarette smoke is a confounding factor, the role of nicotine alone must be addressed. Because human experimentation would be unethical, it is critical to design animal models of fetal nicotine exposure that permit the separation of variables and isolation of the effects of nicotine.

Selection of animal models, doses, and routes of administration

Until the last decade, nearly all investigators used injections of nicotine in pregnant animals as a model for studying fetal development effects. Although bolus nicotine doses cause inappropriately higher peak plasma levels than human smoking, the model is applicable to smoking because the spikes produce episodic ischemia–hypoxia due to the vascular effects of nicotine (Fig. 9-1).[1] However, when the objective is to determine whether nicotine directly affects fetal development, it is better to use implantable minipumps to administer a steady-state nicotine infusion. The infusion model avoids hypoxia–ischemia while permitting fetal exposures at plasma levels of nicotine comparable with those found in typical smokers.[2,3]

Because most studies have been conducted in rats, it is important to determine the appropriate level of exposure in light of species differences in metabolism, pharmacokinetics, and pharmacodynamics of nicotine. The most common dosage used when studying rats, 6 mg/kg/day, may seem unreasonably high on the basis of dose per unit weight. This dose produces plasma levels of nicotine that are approximately double those detected in moderate to heavy smokers.[2] However, in terms of pharmacological effect, the most relevant variable in trying to develop a model that is parallel to humans, it must be kept in mind that the rat is relatively insensitive to nicotine,[4] so that 6 mg/kg/day elicits the electrophysiological changes that reflect nicotine's impact on central nervous system function.[2] A total of 6 mg/kg/day given to pregnant rats also reproduces the fetal growth retardation and fetal resorption seen in fetuses of women who smoke heavily during preg-

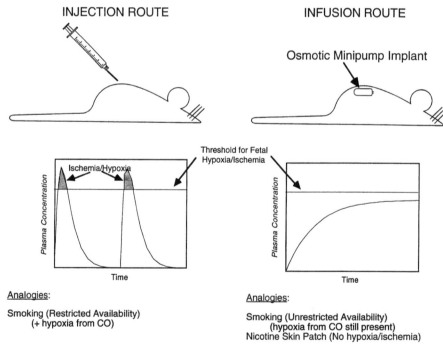

Figure 9-1. Comparison of injection and infusion routes for dosing of pregnant rats with nicotine.

nancy.[1] However, it is important to verify that developmental changes can be detected at lower nicotine exposure levels, such as 2 mg/kg/day, which produce plasma levels comparable with those of human smokers but do not cause fetal growth retardation or resorption in rats.[5]

Nicotine injection model

Daily administration of nicotine subcutaneously to pregnant rats throughout gestation shares numerous features of cigarette smoking, with significant fetal resorption and intrauterine growth retardation accompanying the hypoxia–ischemia experienced with each injection.[6,7] Measurement of sensitive biochemical markers of cell development demonstrates the presence of cell damage, interference with cell replication and growth, and deletion of neurons in favor of glia, a pattern typical of nonspecific injury, such as that elicited by exposure to heavy metals or hypoxia.[1]

At the synaptic level, a number of different transmitter pathways, notably catecholaminergic projections, display hyperactivity consequent to synaptic hyperproliferation in the damaged areas—again, typical of early neuronal injury.[1] Because hypoxia itself can elicit the same effects, it is unlikely that such damage is related to nicotine exposure per se. Hypoxia and ischemia are consequences of human cigarette smoking, and, therefore, these results are relevant to the issue of smoking and fetal brain damage. However, to determine whether nicotine acts on the fetal brain by itself, the infusion model must be employed.

Nicotine infusion model

Administering 6 mg/kg/day of nicotine by continuous infusion throughout gestation, which produces plasma levels of nicotine above those found in smokers, produces many of the adverse effects of smoking during pregnancy, such as fetal resorption and growth retardation.[3,8] However, when the dose is dropped to 2 mg/kg/day, which produces plasma levels comparable with those in moderate smokers, these general toxic effects disappear (reflecting the lowered pharmacological effectiveness of nicotine in rats versus humans).[5] Most importantly, brain cell development is still affected adversely, even with a dose that does not cause growth retardation. The predominant outcomes are interference with neural cell replication and persistently subnormal synaptic activity, despite normal synaptic proliferation—effects that ultimately translate into neuroendocrine and behavioral abnormalities.[1,9,10] In view of the absence of hypoxic–ischemic damage in the infusion model, it is not surprising that the pattern of damage differs from that seen with nicotine injections.

It is particularly notable that the effects of infused nicotine are still prominent, even at doses that do not affect fetal or neonatal growth.[5] This makes nicotine an atypical teratogen because most agents affecting fetal development display brain sparing, wherein the central nervous system is much less affected than the rest of the body. Instead, nicotine targets the brain even when the rest of the organism is spared. The underlying reason is the effects of nicotine on specific neurotransmitter receptors that are present in the fetal nervous system and that normally transduce trophic signals for cell differentiation. Normally, the onset of cholinergic neurotransmission provides the appropriate target cell stimulation, specifically supplying the signal to stop dividing and to proceed with differentiation, axonogenesis, and architectural modeling of brain regions.[11,12] The presence of nicotinic receptors in the fetal brain, well before the natural spike of cholinergic neuronal activity, means that cells exposed to nicotine via the maternal–fetal circulation are receiving the stimulatory signal from the drug during fetal life instead of awaiting the onset of innervation after birth. Consequently, the replication/differentiation switchover is made prematurely, resulting in permanent cell deficits.[12] The best demonstration of this effect is that direct administration of nicotine leads to immediate mitotic arrest, an effect mediated through cholinergic nicotinic receptors and, accordingly, displaying a regional hierarchy corresponding to the concentration of these receptors, namely, midbrain + brainstem ≈ forebrain > cerebellum (Fig. 9-2).[13]

The same effects can be elicited by administering a minute dose of nicotine directly into the cerebrospinal fluid.[13] Chronic administration produces prolonged nicotinic receptor stimulation in the fetal brain and persistent interference with cell replication, as evidenced by the parallel events of upregulation of ^{3}H-

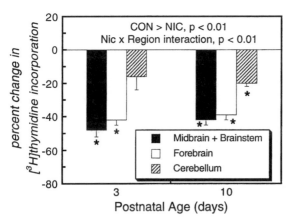

Figure 9-2. Effects of acute nicotine administration on DNA synthesis in developing brain regions, assessed with ^{3}H-thymidine incorporation over a 30-minute period after nicotine Note: The selectivity indicates greater effects in the regions enriched in nicotinic cholinergic receptors (midbrain + brain stem, forebrain) than in a region poor in receptors (cerebellum). (Data from McFarland et al.[13])

nicotine–binding sites, loss of DNA synthetic capability, and the final endpoint of reduced cell numbers, even when the dose of nicotine is restricted to below the threshold for body growth retardation.[3,5]

Nicotine and sudden infant death syndrome

Although a great deal of attention has been paid to nicotine-induced neurobehavioral abnormalities, relatively few studies have addressed the potential role of nicotine in the perinatal morbidity and mortality associated with maternal smoking. Epidemiological studies suggest that maternal smoking accounts for more than 100,000 fetal and perinatal deaths annually in the United States and for a majority of the sudden infant death syndrome (SIDS) cases.[14,15] The relationship between smoking and SIDS is stronger than that seen with any other drugs of abuse and, as a contributing variable, can account for the apparently positive relationships to exposure to other substances.[14] Thus, the same questions need to be answered here as were considered for the effects on brain development, and models of nicotine exposure were applied to that end.[16,17]

SIDS requires the conjunction of two developmental problems: (1) an underlying defect in neonatal cardiovascular and respiratory control and (2) a precipitating event, assumed to be a period of sleep apnea or airway obstruction that produces hypoxia.[18,19] Survival during neonatal hypoxia involves a series of physiological mechanisms that is unique to the developing organism. Among the most important components is the massive release of catecholamines from the adrenal medulla,[20,21] which elicits the required redistribution of blood flow to the brain and heart and maintains cardiac rhythm despite oxygen starvation.[21] One key feature of this reaction is that adrenal catecholamine release is autonomous and occurs independently of central reflexes because of the immaturity of splanchnic innervation.[21]

The persistence of this mechanism into the neonatal period is responsible, in large part, for the ability of the neonate to resist hypoxia. It is, therefore, critically important that prenatal exposure to 6 mg/kg/day of nicotine led to the complete loss of hypoxia-induced adrenomedullary release and to the deaths of a significant number of animals during the hypoxic episode (Fig. 9-3).[16] No increase in hypoxia-induced mortality was seen with 2 mg/kg/day of nicotine, but this finding should be interpreted with caution. If even only a few percent of the animals were to have been sensitized to hypoxia-induced mortality (a proportion that would not be statistically detectable in this experimental design), the same frequency of effect in a large human population would obviously have devastating consequences.

We have also identified the mechanism underlying the defect in adrenomedullary function caused by prenatal nicotine exposure. The adrenal chromaffin cells retain their ability to respond to depolarizing stimuli, and the onset of innervation

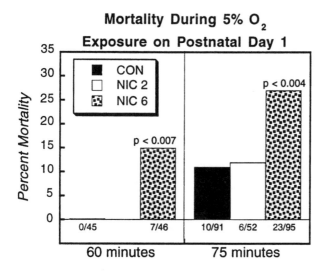

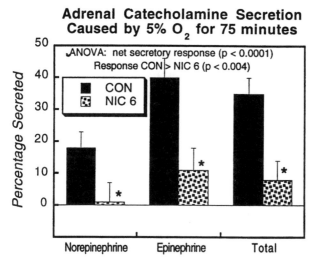

Figure 9-3. Effects of prenatal nicotine exposure at 2 or 6 mg/kg/day on survival during a 60- or 75-minute exposure to hypoxia on postnatal day 1. Note: Numbers at the bottom of each bar represent number dead/number tested. The bottom panel shows the adrenal secretory response to hypoxia. (Data from Slotkin et al.[16])

by the splanchnic nerve is unaffected. Instead, what occurs is quite similar to the mechanism operating in the central nervous system. Because the adrenal chromaffin cells possess nicotinic receptors early in development, stimulation by chronic nicotine exposure accelerates cell differentiation by mimicking the cholinergic trophic signal that would normally arrive with the development of innervation (7–10 days postnatally). The onset of innervation leads to the loss of the unique autonomous response of the adrenal to hypoxia,[21] and, thus, accelerated differentiation leads to premature loss of this mechanism, leaving the animal without protection from hypoxia. That is, the adrenal cannot respond autonomously, and nerve connections are not functional to allow for reflex secretion to take place. Nicotine exposure can thus be viewed as opening up a developmental window of vulnerability to hypoxia in which animals are prone to sudden death.

Two other defects were also identified in the nicotine-exposed animals that could contribute to intolerance to hypoxia. First, biochemical indices indicated that nicotine sensitized cardiac cells to hypoxia, so that each hypoxic episode resulted in increasing degrees of cell injury.[17] Second, we found evidence for dysfunction of central nuclei mediating respiratory control,[16] specifically involving the persistence of fetal response patterns that would produce respiratory arrest during hypoxia (the fetal pattern) as opposed to activation (the postnatal pattern). In this scenario, based on animal models of prenatal nicotine exposure, an exposed infant would be at greater risk for cardiorespiratory failure and death during neonatal apneic episodes as a result of the combined adrenomedullary, cardiac, and respiratory defects.

Conclusions

Animal models of fetal nicotine exposure allow the separation of multiple factors producing structural and functional abnormalities in the offspring of women who smoke. In addition, these models enable us to ascertain the specific roles of nicotine itself. Use of continuous infusions of nicotine throughout gestation has produced results showing that nicotine is a neuroteratogen, leading to the arrest of cell replication and long-term shortfalls of synaptic activity. Importantly, because nicotine acts on specific neurotransmitter receptors, its actions are exerted at doses below the threshold for growth retardation or other general toxicity markers. This distinguishes nicotine from general teratogens, which typically spare the brain relative to the rest of the fetus.

The physiological defects associated with SIDS can be reproduced in animals exposed to nicotine prenatally, providing a mechanistic explanation for the epidemiological association of tobacco use with SIDS. The issue of nicotine administration in a therapeutic setting, either for smoking cessation or as a medication for other medical disorders, remains problematic in considering the potential impact on the fetus. Certainly, a smoker can be encouraged to refrain from smoking and to substitute nicotine to avoid fetal damage associated with the hypoxic–ischemic component of smoking. However, because significant damage can be caused by nicotine itself, many of the basic injurious events may still occur. Furthermore, standard developmental indices of safety, such as fetal or neonatal weight, are inappropriate because the threshold for impaired nervous system development lies below that for growth suppression. If nicotine regimens are chosen that deliver more total nicotine than does smoking, or that allow for greater fetal penetration (steady-state levels maintained around the clock rather than episodic spikes of nicotine during waking hours only), or where occasional smoking continues in the presence of the nicotine substitute, the nicotine-related aspects of fetal nervous system damage may be as bad as or worse than those associated with light or moderate smoking. Nicotine replacement is not likely to provide a panacea to avoid neurobehavioral damage or SIDS in the offspring of smoking mothers. In light of our findings in rats, the only safe course is to discontinue nicotine exposure during pregnancy.

Acknowledgment

This work was supported by a grant from the Smokeless Tobacco Research Council.

References

1. Slotkin TA: Prenatal exposure to nicotine: What can we learn from animal models? In Zagon IS, Slotkin TA (eds): *Maternal Substance Abuse and the Developing Nervous System.* San Diego: Academic Press, 1992, pp. 97–124.
2. Lichtensteiger W, et al.: Prenatal adverse effects of nicotine on the developing brain. *Progress in Brain Research* 1988, 73:137–157.
3. Slotkin TA, et al.: Development of [^{3}H]nicotine binding sites in brain regions of rats exposed to nicotine prenatally via maternal injections or infusions. *Journal of Pharmacology and Experimental Therapeutics* 1987, 242:232–237.
4. Barnes CD, Eltherington LG: *Drug Dosage in Laboratory Animals: A Handbook,* revised ed. Berkeley: University of California Press, 1973.
5. Navarro HA, et al.: Prenatal exposure to nicotine impairs nervous system development at a dose which does not affect viability or growth. *Brain Research Bulletin* 1989, 23:187–192.
6. Slotkin TA, et al.: Effects of prenatal nicotine exposure on neuronal development: Selective actions on central and peripheral catecholaminergic pathways. *Brain Research Bulletin* 1987, 18:601–611.
7. Navarro HA, et al.: Prenatal exposure to nicotine via maternal infusions: Effects on development of catecholamine systems. *Journal of Pharmacology and Experimental Therapeutics* 1988, 244:940–944.
8. Slotkin TA, et al.: Effects of prenatal nicotine exposure on biochemical development of rat brain regions: Maternal drug infusions via osmotic minipumps. *Journal of Pharmacology and Experimental Therapeutics* 1987, 240:602–611.
9. Lichtensteiger W, Schlumpf M: Prenatal nicotine affects fetal testosterone and sexual dimorphism of saccharin preference. *Pharmacology, Biochemistry, and Behavior.* 1985, 23:439–444.
10. Ribary U, Lichtensteiger W: Effects of acute and chronic prenatal nicotine treatment on central catecholamine systems of male and female rat fetuses and offspring. *Journal of Pharmacology and Experimental Therapeutics* 1989, 248:786–792.
11. Hohmann CF, et al.: Neonatal lesions of the basal forebrain cholinergic neurons result in abnormal cortical development. *Developmental Brain Research* 1988, 42:253–264.

12. Navarro HA, et al.: Effects of prenatal nicotine exposure on development of central and peripheral cholinergic neurotransmitter systems. Evidence for cholinergic trophic influences in developing brain. *Journal of Pharmacology and Experimental Therapeutics* 1989, 251:894–900.

13. McFarland BJ, et al.: Inhibition of DNA synthesis in neonatal rat brain regions caused by acute nicotine administration. *Developmental Brain Research* 1991, 58:223–229.

14. Haglund B, Cnattingius S: Cigarette smoking as a risk factor for sudden infant death syndrome: A population-based study. *American Journal of Public Health* 1990, 80: 29–32.

15. DiFranza JR, Lew RA: Effect of maternal cigarette smoking on pregnancy complications and sudden infant death syndrome. *Journal of Family Practice* 1995, 40: 385–394.

16. Slotkin TA, et al.: Loss of neonatal hypoxia tolerance after prenatal nicotine exposure: Implications for sudden infant death syndrome. *Brain Research Bulletin* 1995, 38: 69–75.

17. Tolson CM, et al.: Do concurrent or prior nicotine exposures interact with neonatal hypoxia to produce cardiac cell damage? *Teratology* 1995, 52:298–305.

18. Stramba-Badiale M, et al.: Development of cardiac innervation, ventricular fibrillation, and sudden infant death syndrome. *American Journal of Physiology* 1992, 263: H1514–H1522.

19. Poets CF, et al.: The relationship between bradycardia, apnea, and hypoxemia in preterm infants. *Pediatric Research* 1993, 34:144–147.

20. Lagercrantz H, Bistoletti P: Catecholamine release in the newborn infant at birth. *Pediatric Research* 1973, 11:889–893.

21. Slotkin TA, Seidler FJ: Adrenomedullary catecholamine release in the fetus and newborn: Secretory mechanisms and their role in stress and survival. *Journal of Developmental Physiology* 1988, 10:1–16.

Chapter 10

Measuring Fetal Exposure to Nicotine

GIDEON KOREN, CHRISOULA ELIOPOULOS, and JULIA KLEIN

In North America, approximately 30% of women 18 years old and older are regular cigarette smokers.[1,2] Nearly half of all pregnancies are unplanned. This means that many women will conceive while smoking, and approximately 60% of women who smoke before pregnancy continue to smoke during pregnancy.[3–5] Since the fetus of a smoking mother is exposed to tobacco smoke, the fetus is a passive smoker.

Nicotine replacement for smoking cessation has to be considered in the context of benefit versus risk. The efficacy of nicotine replacement in the treatment of smoking cessation has been repeatedly proven. Exposing women to nicotine in a replacement therapy in amounts equal to or lower than what they had consumed with cigarette smoking should not increase fetal risk. Because animal studies suggest that nicotine by itself may induce fetal neurotoxicity, however, replacing cigarette smoke with nicotine may not ensure reasonable fetal safety. Thus, it may be advisable for pregnant women, or women planning pregnancy, to undergo a pharmacokinetic study measuring their blood cotinine levels before nicotine replacement therapy, thus establishing an optimal ethical solution for future uses of nicotine replacement therapy for pregnant women.

Currently, investigators rely primarily on maternal self-reports to assess gestational tobacco exposure. However, this method is not very reliable. Smoking behavior varies during pregnancy. Thus, a single interview with a pregnant woman may not adequately reflect the variability in smoke exposure over the course of her pregnancy, and some women may not disclose their smoking habits.[6] Clearly, an objective measure of cigarette smoking, accounting for parameters other than the claimed number of cigarettes smoked, is needed. To date, the presence and level of nicotine in the body is the most specific measure of exposure to cigarette smoke.[7,8]

There is a correlation between maternal and neonatal concentrations of nicotine and cotinine, which cross the placenta in a predictable manner. Nicotine and cotinine have been found in hair, allowing for assessment of long-term cigarette smoke exposure. However, investigations involving this technique have been lacking.

The Toronto Study

The Toronto Study researchers developed a way to measure drug histories by examining hair content.[9] Two main objectives were identified for study: (1) comparing hair analysis of nicotine and cotinine with maternal self-reported exposure to cigarette smoke and (2) investigating the relationship between maternal reports or hair nicotine and cotinine concentrations with pregnancy outcome measurements. Hair concentration provides a long-term history of drug use because drugs are deposited into the hair shaft and grow with it. Based on typical hair growth rates, drug use can be estimated by evaluating segments of hair. Between September and December 1992, one investigator attended the newborn nursery at the Toronto Hospital, General Division, Toronto, Ontario, three times a week to enroll study participants. All mothers were asked to complete a brief questionnaire detailing their smoking habits. At this time, maternal and neonatal hair samples were collected from each enrolled mother–infant pair.

A recent report of this cohort showed that infants of passive smokers had significantly higher amounts of cotinine in their hair at birth than infants of nonsmokers.[9] This analysis also revealed that infants prenatally exposed to both maternal and paternal smoking had higher levels of cotinine in their hair than infants exposed to maternal smoking alone. Although there was a distinction in amounts of cotinine in hair between infants of passive smokers and active smokers, a significant difference was not seen when infants of passive smokers were compared with infants of a subgroup of women who smoked but were not exposed to passive smoke. More than 50% of the smokers in this study were light smokers. Overlapping urinary cotinine values between passive smokers and light smokers have been previously reported. Thus, consistent exposure to second-hand smoke may not be that different from light smoking.

Collection and analysis of samples

Clinical data collected included the average number of cigarettes smoked and exposure to passive smoke during each trimester. Subjects were identified as active smokers, passive smokers, or nonsmokers. Active smokers were defined as women who admitted smoking cigarettes at any time during their pregnancies.

Active smokers were then subdivided into two groups: (1) those who lived or worked with other smokers and (2) those who were exposed only to their own smoking. Passive smokers were defined as nonsmoking women who were exposed to other persons' smoke for at least 2 hours a day throughout pregnancy. Women classified as nonsmokers reported no regular exposure to cigarette smoke during pregnancy. Maternal data collected included date of birth, race, marital status, obstetric history, maternal diseases, and medication.

Data retrieved from the neonatal charts included sex, date of birth, method of delivery, gestational age, birth weight, head circumference, birth length, presence or absence of meconium at delivery, method of resuscitation, special-care requirements, and congenital malformations. Resuscitation was categorized as spontaneous or supportive. Resuscitation was considered supportive in cases where newborns required oxygen stimulation, oxygen bagging, oxygen suction, oxygen by mask, endotracheal tube and suction, oropharyngeal suctioning, bulb suctioning, or tracheal aspiration at delivery. Infants admitted to the neonatal intensive care unit were classified as requiring special care.

Hair samples from the mother–infant pairs were obtained by cutting 20–25 hair shafts from mothers and 5–7 from their infants. The longest hair from the occipital region of the scalp was obtained from neonates because this may represent the earliest development of scalp hair.[10] This area is generally chosen for hair sampling as most of the hair in this region is in the anagen phase of growth.[11] All hair samples were collected 1–3 days following delivery. The following day, hair was tested to determine the average content of nicotine or cotinine. The results were expressed as nanograms of nicotine or cotinine per milligram of hair.

Washing conditions to remove sources of external contamination, without removing systemically deposited drugs in hair, are not standardized across studies. Various washing regimens have been employed,[12–17] but there has been some debate as to whether some of the solvents used may be too stringent and remove systemically deposited drugs.[18] Thus, some investigators have not washed hair at all. In the Toronto study, shampoo was used to remove contamination as it does not strip deposited drugs from hair strands.

Data analysis

The total nicotine content in hair has been shown to be directly proportional to both the air concentration of nicotine and the duration of exposure.[19] This fact may account for large nicotine-to-cotinine ratios observed in maternal hair samples. External contamination is less of a problem with analysis of hair for cotinine because it is derived from hepatic metabolism, and, thus, its route of entry into hair is through the systemic circulation. Hair obtained from neonates shortly after birth is unlikely to be externally contaminated by environmental tobacco smoke. This is indicated by the smaller nicotine-to-cotinine ratios observed in neonatal hair samples.

Cotinine has a much longer elimination half-life than nicotine, and self-reported smoking habits have been better validated by measurements of this metabolite in plasma, urine, and saliva.[7,8,12,20,21] Thus, cotinine levels in hair should be more sensitive than nicotine in distinguishing between different groups of smoke-exposed infants.[9] To date, no other studies have assessed cotinine levels in neonatal hair. Previous studies assessing adult hair have demonstrated that cotinine concentrations in the hair of nonsmokers ranges from 0 to 0.4 ng/mg hair, with a mean of 0.1 ng/mg hair.[22,23] Kintz et al.[23] reported that the range of cotinine in the hair of passive smokers and nonsmokers is the same. Thus, the sample size was calculated so that a twofold difference in the hair levels of cotinine could be detected between infants of passive smokers and nonsmokers.

Correlations between maternal and neonatal hair concentrations of nicotine and cotinine, and between the number of cigarettes smoked and hair measurements, were studied by least-square regression analysis for data that were normally distributed. Logarithmic transformation of the data or Spearman's rank correlation coefficient was used to compare nonparametric data.

Misclassification of active smokers or nonsmokers due to undisclosed smoking cannot be ruled out. Passive smokers may be misclassified as nonsmokers because of significant exposure not accounted for by the questionnaire. The true difference in neonatal hair concentrations may have been diluted, and hair accumulation of cotinine in passive smokers may be higher. These findings have been supported by Ostrea and colleagues.[24] In the Ostrea et al. examination of meconium for cotinine content, cotinine levels among passive smokers were found to be higher than the levels seen with nonsmokers.

In a study by Pley et al.,[25] recall bias was demonstrated by having women record the number of cigarettes they smoked per day during pregnancy. A subsequent review indicated under-reporting of smoking. It is recognized that under-reporting of smoking is common among groups that perceive admitting (e.g. to a physician who has advised that one quit smoking) smoking as undesirable.[25]

Maternal characteristics and reported exposure to cigarette smoke

The majority of smoking women were light to moderate smokers, yet there was a great degree of variability in the amount of nicotine and cotinine extracted from hair in these women and their infants. This may be attributed to the fact that the number of cigarettes smoked is only one determinant of systemic exposure. Individual differences in tobacco smoke uptake (i.e., the way a cigarette is smoked) and metabolism are additional factors for consideration. Indeed, the sum of these individual factors determines total systemic maternal and fetal exposure to cigarette smoke as is evidenced by the excellent correlation between maternal and neonatal hair levels of cotinine.

A total of 93 mothers and their newborns were included in this study. Of these subjects, 36 were classified as active smokers, 22 were passive smokers, and 35

were nonsmokers. One passive-smoking woman delivered twins, leading to a total of 94 mother–infant pairs. The mean age of these women was 31 years, and
ages ranged from 17 to 43 years. There was no difference in age or ethnicity between active, passive, and nonsmoking women in this study.

Among the 36 active smokers, 4 women quit smoking within the first trimester
of pregnancy. A total of 20 women reported that they were the only smoker in
their household; 16 stated that they lived with a smoker (in most cases, their
spouse). The mean number of cigarettes smoked each day was approximately 12
and ranged from 1 to 40 cigarettes per day. A total of 58% of the smoking women
smoked from 1 to 10 cigarettes per day. Few women studied were heavy smokers;
only 1 of the 36 women smoked more than 25 cigarettes per day. Among the 22
women who reported passive exposure to cigarette smoke, 21 identified the primary source of exposure to be from home.

Neonatal characteristics

A total of 55 male and 39 female infants were enrolled in this study. Gestational
age ranged from 31 to 43 weeks; birth weights ranged from 2,040 to 4,460 g. The
three groups of infants did not differ with respect to gender, age, head circumference, or Apgar scores at 1 and 5 minutes of life. A significant decrease in mean
birth weight was observed for those infants born to smokers even after controlling
for gestational age. Infants of smokers had significantly shorter mean lengths
than infants of passive smokers and nonsmokers.

Three low-birth-weight infants (weighing less than 2,500 g) were identified in
this study population, and they were all born to smoking women. Five of six premature infants (born before 37 weeks of gestation) were born to smoking women;
one premature infant was born to a passive smoker. Thirteen of the infants enrolled in this study were admitted into the neonatal intensive care unit for care.
There were significantly more cases requiring attention in the neonatal intensive
care unit among active smokers ($n = 10$) than passive smokers ($n = 2$) and nonsmokers ($n = 1$) ($p < 0.01$). Among active smokers, there were two cases of opioid withdrawal and six of respiratory distress. With respect to congenital abnormalities, three were described among the smoking women: one sacrococcygeal
teratoma, one right kidney agenesis, and one left ear anomaly. Among the passive
smoking women, one infant was born with a genital hydrocoele. Among the nonsmoking women, one infant was born with hypospadias.

Maternal and neonatal hair concentrations of nicotine and cotinine

Preliminary results of the Toronto Study have been published.[9] Among the smoking women, there was no significant difference observed in hair levels of nicotine

or cotinine between women who were the only smokers in their households and women who smoked in addition to other household members.

Among the subgroups of smokers, infants born to women who smoked with other household smokers had significantly greater levels of cotinine in their hair than infants of women who smoked alone. Hair concentrations of cotinine were not different between infants of women who smoked alone and those of passive smoking women.

Small amounts of nicotine and cotinine were detected in the hair of nonsmokers and their infants. This is not surprising as small amounts of nicotine are present in common foods such as potatoes, tomatoes, eggplants, and teas.[26] Also, cigarette smoke in the environment is ubiquitous, considering that more than 30% of Canadians are regular smokers. Despite uncontrolled sources of exposure, the relatively different concentrations of cotinine in hair allowed for distinctions between different groups of cigarette-smoke–exposed infants.

Conclusions

Nicotine and cotinine levels can be accurately measured in the hair of neonates and their mothers. With the availability of smoking cessation aids such as nicotine replacement therapy, physicians are presented with an opportunity to help pregnant smoking women quit smoking. However, delivering nicotine to pregnant women presents an ethical dilemma. On the one hand, smoking cessation is more probable if nicotine replacement therapy is used; on the other hand, nicotine can have adverse effects on fetuses. The ethical dilemma can, however, be resolved if an accurate level of maternal self-administration of nicotine can be obtained. Provided that an accurate level is obtained prior to administration of nicotine replacement therapy, and nicotine is delivered in doses that do not exceed the maternal self-administered amounts, the most ethical treatment can be to administer nicotine because the chances of success in smoking cessation are much greater if a nicotine replacement therapy is used. Because hair can be assessed for nicotine levels over time, hair measurement of nicotine and cotinine levels is an excellent method for obtaining the baseline values needed to determine the amount of nicotine advisable to deliver as part of a smoking cessation program.

Acknowledgement

This work was supported by a grant from the Medical Research Council of Canada.

References

1. Stachenko SJ, Reeder BA, Lindsay E, Donovan C, Lessard R, Balram C: Smoking prevalence and associated risk factors in Canadian adults. *Canadian Medical Association Journal* 1992, 146:1989–1996.

2. Williamson DF, Serdula MK, Kendrick JS, Binkin NJ: Comparing the prevalence of smoking in pregnant and nonpregnant women, 1985–1986. *Journal of the American Medical Association* 1989, 261:70–74.
3. Stewart PJ, Dunkley GC: Smoking and health care patterns among pregnant women. *Canadian Medical Association Journal* 1985, 133:989–994.
4. Fingerhut LA, Kleinman JC, Kendrick JS: Smoking before, during, and after pregnancy. *American Journal of Public Health* 1990, 80:541–544.
5. O'Campo R, Faden RR, Brown H, Gielen AC: The impact of pregnancy on women's prenatal and postpartum smoking behavior. *American Journal of Preventive Medicine* 1992, 8:8–13.
6. Mullen PD, Carbonari JP, Tabak ER, Glenday MC: Improving disclosure of smoking by pregnant women. *American Journal of Obstetrics and Gynecology* 1991, 165: 409–413.
7. Muranka H, Higashi E, Itani S, Shimizu Y: Evaluation of nicotine, cotinine, thiocyanate, carboxyhemoglobin, and expired carbon monoxide as biochemical tobacco smoke uptake parameters. *International Archives of Occpational and Environmental Health* 1988, 60:37–41.
8. Jarvis MJ, Tunstall-Pedoe H, Feyerabend C, Vesey C, Saloojee Y: Comparison of tests to distinguish smokers from nonsmokers. *American Journal of Public Health* 1987, 77:1435–1438.
9. Eliopoulos C, Klein J, Khan Phan M, Knie B, Greenwald M, Chitayat D, Koren G: Hair concentrations of nicotine and cotinine in women and their newborn infants. *Journal of the American Medical Association* 1994, 271:621–623.
10. Pecoraro V, Astore IPL: Measurements of hair growth under physiological conditions. In Orfanos CE, Happle R (eds): *Hair and Hair Diseases*. New York: Springer-Verlag, 1990, pp 237–254.
11. Forslind B: The growing anagen hair. In Orfanos CE, Happle R (eds): *Hair and Hair Diseases*. New York: Springer-Verlag, 1990, pp 73–97.
12. Haley NJ, Axelrad CM, Tilton KA: Validation of self-reported smoking behavior: Biochemical analyses of cotinine and thiocyanate. *American Journal of Public Health* 1983, 73:1204–1207.
13. Baumgartner W, Hill VA, Blahd WH: Hair analysis for drugs of abuse. *Journal of Forensic Science* 1989, 34:1433–1453.
14. Ishiyama I, Nagai T, Toshida S: Detection of basic drugs (methamphetamine, antidepressants, and nicotine) from human hair. *Journal of Forensic Science* 1983, 28: 380–385.
15. Mizuno A, Uematsu T, Oshima A, Nakamura M, Nakashima M: Analysis of nicotine content of hair for assessing individual cigarette-smoking behavior. *Therapeutic Drug Monitor* 1993, 15:99–104.
16. Kintz P, Mangin P: Hair analysis for detection of beta-blockers in hypertensive patients. *European Journal of Clinical Pharmacology* 1992, 42:351–352.
17. Bost RO: Hair analysis—Perspectives and limits of a proposed forensic method of proof: A review. *Forensic Science International* 1993, 93:31–42.
18. Langone JJ, Gjika HB, Van Vunakis H: Nicotine and its metabolites. Radioimmunoassays for nicotine and cotinine. *Biochemistry* 1973, 12:5025–5030.
19. Nilsen T, Zahlsen K, Nilsen OG: Uptake of nicotine in hair during controlled environmental air exposure to nicotine vapor: Evidence for a major contribution of environmental nicotine to overall nicotine found in hair from smokers and non-smokers. *Pharmacological Toxicology* 1994, 75:136–142.

20. Greenberg RA, Haley NJ, Etzel RA, Loda FA: Measuring the exposure of infants to tobacco smoke. Nicotine and cotinine in urine and saliva. *New England Journal of Medicine* 1984, 310:1075–1078.
21. Haley NJ, Hoffmann D: Analysis for nicotine and cotinine in hair to determine cigarette smoker status. *Clinical Chemistry* 1985, 31:1598–1600.
22. Rosa M, Pacifici R, Altieri I, Pichini S, Ottaviani G, Zuccaro P: How the steady-state cotinine concentration in cigarette smokers is directly related to nicotine intake. *Clinical Pharmacology and Therapeutics* 1992, 52:324–329.
23. Kintz P, Ludes B, Mangin P: Evaluation of nicotine and cotinine in human hair. *Journal of Forensic Science* 1992, 37:72–76.
24. Ostrea EM, Knapp DK, Romero A, Montes M, Ostrea AR: Meconium analysis to assess fetal exposure to nicotine by active and passive maternal smoking. *Journal of Pediatrics* 1994, 124:471–476.
25. Pley EAP, Wouters EJM, Voohorst FJ, Stolte SB, Kurver PHJ, de Jong PA: Assessment of tobacco-exposure during pregnancy; behavioral and biochemical changes. *European Journal of Obstetrics, Gynecology, and Reproductive Biology* 1991, 40: 197–201.
26. Davis RA, Stiles MF, DeBethizy JD, Reynolds JH: Dietary nicotine: A source of urinary cotinine. *Food and Chemical Toxicology* 1991, 29:821–827.

Chapter 11

Human Studies of Nicotine Replacement During Pregnancy

CHERYL A. ONCKEN, HILDUR HARDARDOTTIR,
and JAMES S. SMELTZER

Nicotine replacement products are currently the most effective pharmacological agents to aid in smoking cessation.[1] A down-rating of nicotine gum and transdermal nicotine by the Food and Drug Administration from category X to categories C and D, respectively, increases the availability of these products to pregnant women.

There are few safety, and no efficacy, data on the use of nicotine replacement products by pregnant women. Nicotine replacement therapy is likely less harmful than smoking during pregnancy because of a lower total nicotine dose, and absence of exposure to carbon monoxide and other toxic substances.[2] Nicotine may be harmful to the developing fetus, given the known risks of smoking during pregnancy[3] and similar effects of pure nicotine administration to pregnant animals.[4]

This chapter seeks to elucidate the known effects and potential toxicity of nicotine in pregnancy by reviewing tobacco-related disturbances and studies of nicotine administration in animals and humans. There is a large species variation in the toxicity and effects of nicotine, so extrapolation from animal studies to humans should be done with caution. However, animal studies do give some insight into the effects of nicotine during pregnancy. Implications of these data are related to nicotine replacement therapy.

Teratogenic effects

During primary organogenesis, a single exposure to a teratogen can produce death or persistent harm to a developing organism. Teratogenic potential is rightly the greatest concern regarding drug administration during pregnancy. Classic teratogenesis occurs in the first trimester, beginning around the date of missed menses, resulting in congenital malformations. This occurs with drugs such as thalidomide, ethanol, and retinoic acid. Smoking has not been consistently associated with congenital malformations in the developing fetus in animal or human studies,[5] despite many exposures. It is unlikely that nicotine replacement can cause a significant increase in frequency of all, or specific, congenital malformations.

Besides congenital malformations, the final manifestations of teratogenesis are growth retardation, functional disorder, and death.[6] In this context, smoking and nicotine are probably teratogenic.

An increased risk of spontaneous abortion is consistently found among smokers.[7] These abortuses are chromosomally normal.[8] Although the mechanism is unknown, nicotine may be the agent. In rats, increased embryonic resorptions[9] and maturation delay occur with nicotine alone.[10]

Each organ undergoes primary organogenesis at different times. Unlike all other organs, which complete organogenesis during the first trimester, the nervous system in humans continues in primary organogenesis well after birth.[11] Nicotinic-binding sites increase in the human fetal brain from 12 to 19 weeks of gestation.[12] High levels of ^{3}H-nicotine-binding sites are found in the human brain stem tegmentum at midgestation, and the profile rapidly changes over at mid to late gestation.[13] Exogenous nicotine administration by any route can potentially alter this development. Research indicating neurotoxic effects of nicotine during this period, and relation of these changes to long-term neurobehavioral effects and sudden infant death syndrome are reviewed in Chapter 9.

The 24-hour transdermal nicotine systems result in continuous nicotine exposure. Concentrations of nicotine in the blood of such patch users at night can exceed those found in smokers. It is unknown if continuous exposure to nicotine has a different effect on the developing fetal brain than intermittent exposure.

Fetal growth

Fetal growth restriction is strongly associated with smoking during pregnancy, with a relative risk of 2.41.[14] Impaired growth is dose dependent and correlates well with serum cotinine concentrations.[15] This growth restriction is symmetrical (head and abdomen are equally influenced), indicating an effect on cell number.[16] Growth restriction is not observed when smoking is discontinued prior to 16 weeks of gestation. [17,18] Fetuses of smoking mothers fail to show "catch-up" growth.[19] Together, these data indicate a continued and cumulative ongoing toxic action.

Animal studies indicate that pure nicotine administration causes growth restriction similar to that seen during smoking and human pregnancy. The guinea pig is a good model with which to study effects on growth because guinea pigs have a hemochorial placenta and their fetal fat composition and growth pattern are more similar to those of humans than are those of rodents. Nicotine administration of 6 mg/kg/day to pregnant guinea pigs throughout gestation results in decreased birth weight and head diameter,[20] which is similar to the pattern observed in humans.[14] Nicotine may also have indirect effects on fetal growth by reducing essential amino acid transport across the placenta by cholinergic blockade.[21]

Growth restriction is related to dose of nicotine in animals and cigarette consumption in humans. A direct toxic effect of nicotine is probable. Therefore, total nicotine exposure during replacement therapy, as reflected by serum cotinine level, should be equivalent to or less than exposure during smoking.

Placental hemodynamics

The placenta has two separate circulations (maternal–uterine and fetal–umbilical) that become contiguous for gas and nutrient exchange. Blood flow in both circulations is near maximal, and blood flow is directly proportional to blood pressure. Although a reduction of blood flow in either circulation could compromise oxygen delivery to the fetus, there is normally an excess of flow over fetal needs. Fetal gas and substrate delivery rates and concentrations are usually preserved even with extended reductions in blood flow.[22]

Other tissues adapt local perfusion to local needs by changing resistance at the level of the end arteriole. The placenta is unique because it is generally unable to increase local blood flow. Before week 20 of human gestation, the trophoblast invades and destroys the muscularis of the maternal arterioles that feed it. This removes the primary control system, which is operative in all other circulations.[23] On the fetal side, placental vessels are near maximal dilation. Therefore, the tone of the feeding arteries (uterine and umbilical) is the major regulator of blood flow to the developing fetus. Moreover, as reviewed by Ford,[24] the uterine artery during pregnancy has other unique properties. There is a proliferation of α_1-adrenergic receptors and hypersensitivity of this circulation to catecholamines.

Maternal placental perfusion

The welfare of the fetus depends on adequate bathing of the chorionic villi by maternal blood. Nicotine may play a role in growth restriction, preterm labor, and stillbirth by reducing maternal uteroplacental blood flow and oxygen delivery acutely. This produces fetal hypoxemia if it exceeds placental reserve and acidosis if it persists.

There is considerable evidence that smoking decreases uteroplacental blood flow. Radioisotope studies show that smoking acutely decreases blood flow[25] with a return to baseline within 15 minutes.[26] One study showed a lower conversion of dehydroepiandrosterone sulfate (DHA-S) to estradiol actutely after smoking, which may indicate impairment of uteroplacental blood flow.[27] Placental pathology of smokers is consistent with intermittent hypoperfusion from the maternal circulation.[28]

Nicotine's effect on uteroplacental blood flow may be dose dependent. Maternal smoking and nicotine administration increase maternal blood pressure, which should increase uteroplacental blood flow. However, either a direct action of nicotine or, more likely, release of circulating catecholamines can result in a significant decrease in uterine perfusion, despite maternal hypertension. A dose-dependent increase, then decrease, in uterine blood flow was found in one sheep study.[29]

Findings in the sheep study may explain conflicting results in studies of the effects of smoking and nicotine on blood flow in humans. Most studies show that smoking acutely reduces uterine blood flow; however, uterine blood flow (measured by Doppler) has, in other studies, been shown to increase after smoking.[30] Other studies failed to find evidence of decreased uterine[31] or fetoplacental[32] blood flow with smoking or 4 mg nicotine gum. With the gum, no increase in circulating epinephrine or norepinephrine concentration was noted.

There appears to be considerable individual variation in the responses of uterine blood flow to smoking one standard cigarette.[26] Variation may be attributable to differential susceptibility or response to adrenergic stimulation. It is clear that most of the hemodynamic effects of smoking in pregnancy are caused by nicotine.[33]

Despite conflicting studies of the effects of lower doses of nicotine administration during pregnancy on blood flow, high doses of intravenous nicotine (14–32 µg/kg body weight per minute in sheep and 1 mg/kg body weight in rhesus monkeys) invariably reduced uterine blood flow[34] and caused hypoxemia and acidosis.[35] Catecholamine release is the likely mechanism by which nicotine mediates a reduction in uterine blood flow in sheep—an action blocked by phentolamine. The reduction in uteroplacental blood flow in the ewe was not observed at nicotine concentrations that did not increase plasma catecholamines.[36]

During pregnancy, circulating catecholamines increase after smoking.[37] Based on animal studies and on the known hyper-responsiveness of the uterine artery to catecholamines, it seems probable that a less deleterious effect on blood flow would be expected with nicotine replacement products than with smoking because the gradual release of nicotine may elicit less adrenal response. A lesser effect on catecholamine release for transdermal nicotine compared with cigarette smoking has been demonstrated in nonpregnant individuals.[38] Data from transdermal nicotine studies evaluating uteroplacental blood flow and catecholamine metabolites are not yet available, but may be informative.

Fetoplacental blood flow

A reduction in fetal blood supply (umbilical blood flow) could also alter oxygen delivery to the fetus. Changes in fetal heart rate and its variability[39] and umbilical blood flow[40] have been frequently found in studies of cigarette smoking and nicotine use in pregnancy. One study, using massive doses of nicotine in the rhesus monkey mother, confirmed fetal hypoxia and acidosis.[35] Other studies, using more typical doses, have not found changes. At concentrations consistent with smoking, a more plausible explanation for changes in fetal heart rate and variability is the direct action of transplacental nicotine on the fetus, with fetal adrenergic stimulation and hypertension.[40]

An in vitro study demonstrated a dose-dependent contraction of the human umbilical artery when exposed to nicotine at concentrations two to four times those seen with cigarette smoking and transdermal nicotine use.[41] Preliminary research does not find such an effect with moderate smoking or with chewing nicotine gum.[32] One study in sheep[42] found an increase in umbilical artery resistance and high stillbirth rate with nicotine administration late in gestation. Another study found a decrease in umbilical blood flow, but only with their highest nicotine doses, in the maternal ewe.[29] Human studies have found an increase in umbilical blood flow.[32,40] Interestingly, the data do not show any compensatory fall in cerebral artery resistance typically found in hypoxia.[42]

Fetal behavioral states

Nicotine may influence fetal behavior such as fetal breathing, movements, and tone. Fetal breathing is a sign of fetal well-being. Reduction in fetal breathing may be caused by hypoxia, central effects, fetal infection, or labor. A bolus intravenous injection of 0.14–0.25 mg/kg nicotine reduced fetal breathing in pregnant ewes.[43] Interestingly, the reduction in fetal breathing did not occur in pregnant ewes when pretreated with phentolamine or when nicotine was infused slowly over 30 minutes, indicating that this effect is mediated by catecholamines. Direct administration of nicotine into the fetal lamb circulation results in increased fetal breathing. These studies suggest that reduction in fetal breathing in animals is caused by hypoxia. The hypoxia appears to be from a reduction in uterine blood flow with catecholamine release in the maternal circulation.

A reduction in fetal breathing also occurs after smoking in humans[44] and has been shown to be secondary to nicotine.[45] Whether the reduction in fetal breathing seen in the human fetus is a result of hypoxia is unknown, but seems probable.

Placental effects

The second strongest epidemiological association of maternal smoking is the incidence of problems related to placentation: abruption (early separation of the normally located placenta) and placenta previa (abnormal location of the placenta). These conditions contribute to the increased prematurity and fetal death rates associated with cigarette smoking and possibly to miscarriage rates.

Smoking and nicotine both acutely increase maternal blood pressure. Unlike other vascular beds, there is no end-arteriolar protection of the uteroplacental circulation from maternal hypertension. Hypertension is the single most important risk factor for placental abruption. There is also increased acute inflammatory changes and necrosis of the decidua basalis at the margin of the placenta in smokers.[28] It seems possible that areas of decidual necrosis may play a role in placental abruption by serving as a nidus for starting dissection and hemorrhage. This would produce further thrombus formation, necrosis, and shearing of the placental bed, producing clinical placental abruption.

If smoking is associated with placental abruption, because of acute rises in maternal blood pressure, the differing effects of smoking and nicotine replacement products would depend on how they acutely increase maternal blood pressure.

Coagulation

Cigarette smoking is associated with an increased risk of coronary artery disease and stroke, and a likely mechanism is activation of coagulation.[46] Thromboxane is a potent vasoconstrictor and coagulant released by cigarette smoking and possibly nicotine administration. Surprisingly, the placentas of smokers have decreased thrombosis of the maternal vessels compared with nonsmokers.[28] This is consistent with epidemiological studies that show smokers have a lower risk of pre-eclampsia than nonsmokers.[47] The reason for this paradoxical finding is unknown, but indicates that placental thrombosis is not a plausible mechanism by which smoking contributes to growth retardation.

Nicotine can also inhibit the production of prostacyclin, an inhibitor of platelet aggregation and potent vasodilator of the umbilical arteries.[48] This could produce deleterious effects on fetoplacental blood flow.

Human studies of nicotine replacement during pregnancy

The effects of single-dose nicotine gum on maternal–fetal hemodynamic parameters have been studied. Collectively, studies show that nicotine alters maternal–fetal hemodynamics during human pregnancy. Nicotine gum (4 or 8 mg), when chewed as a single dose, reduces fetal breathing,[44] and 2 mg nicotine gum alters fetal heart rate variability[39] (postulated secondary to either fetal adrenergic stimulation or hypoxemia or both). Nicotine increases blood flow in the fetoplacental circulation when catecholamines are not effected.[32] In nearly all of these studies, the fetal effects of nicotine are dose related.

We conducted a prospective, randomized study to compare the safety and effects of continued gum chewing versus smoking during anticipated steady-state conditions.[49] Study subjects were randomized to continue smoking or to quit smoking and chew 2 mg nicotine gum ad libitum for 5 days. We found that the overall nicotine exposure, as measured by plasma cotinine level, was significantly less with gum chewing than with continued smoking. In addition, peak and trough nicotine concentrations and hemodynamic effects were generally less with gum use than with continued smoking. This study indicates that short-term nicotine gum use is likely safer than smoking in pregnant smokers unable to quit without such measures.

Implications for nicotine replacement during pregnancy

There is no known safe dose of nicotine that can be administered during pregnancy. It is clear from the previous discussion that nicotine can cause fetal harm by multiple mechanisms. Thus, nicotine replacement should be considered if the likelihood of smoking cessation appears low without such measures.

Because many of the effects of smoking during pregnancy are dose related, nicotine replacement should only be offered if it delivers equivalent or lower concentrations of nicotine than are usually achieved with smoking. Nicotine gum provides lower doses, and transdermal nicotine use during pregnancy is currently being studied. Use of nasal spray and vapor inhalation during pregnancy has not been studied.

Multiple animal studies suggest that reduction in uterine blood flow, which occurs during peak nicotine concentration, results from catecholamine release. Thus, it seems plausible that the pharmacodynamic effects of a nicotine bolus, as with smoking, are likely to have a more deleterious effect on uteroplacental blood flow than sustained release nicotine (gum and patch). A chronic effect of nicotine on uterine blood flow cannot be excluded, however. This is currently being studied in pregnant smokers.

Data support better pregnancy outcomes with earlier smoking cessation. If smoking is discontinued prior to 16 weeks of gestation, then much of the growth restriction can be avoided. Mid to late gestation appears to be the period most vulnerable to the harmful effects of nicotine for the developing human fetal brain.[13] Thus, during pregnancy, the goal is to be smoke and nicotine free, especially during the third trimester. The mature fetus responds more adversely to nicotine administration than does the immature fetus. If it is necessary to begin nicotine replacement therapy, the sooner used and discontinued, the better, if the result is smoking cessation.

The safety of transdermal nicotine usage during pregnancy has not been established. Until definitive answers are found, potential neurotoxicity of continuous exposure should preclude general, 24-hour usage at this time.

Conclusions

Current data are sufficient to indicate that a rule-of-thumb approach is justified: Nicotine replacement therapy can be considered reasonably safe only to the extent that it does not exceed the physiological perturbations or fetoplacental nicotine exposure of the pre-existing smoking behavior it treats. Efficacy in pregnancy currently cannot be addressed. Clearly, nicotine exposure may be harmful during pregnancy, and, while nicotine replacement therapy is probably less harmful than smoking, there is no safe dose of nicotine during pregnancy. Therefore, efficacy should be measured by proven reduction in exposure of mother and fetus to nicotine.

Acknowledgments

This chapter was supported in part by NIH General Clinical Research Center grant M01RR06192.

References

1. Henningfield JE: Drug therapy: Nicotine medications for smoking cessation. *New England Journal of Medicine* 1995, 333:1196–1203.
2. Benowitz N: Nicotine replacement therapy during pregnancy. *Journal of the American Medical Association* 1991, 266:3174–3177.
3. Floyd RL, Rimer BK, Giovino GA, Mullen PD, Sullivan SE: A review of smoking in pregnancy: Effects on pregnancy outcomes and cessation efforts. *Annual Review of Public Health* 1993, 14:379–411.
4. Abel EL: Smoking during pregnancy: A review of effects on growth and development of offspring. *Human Biology* 1980, 52:593–625.
5. Werler MM, Pober BR, Holmes LB: Smoking and pregnancy. *Teratology* 1985, 32: 473–481.
6. Wilson JG: Current status of teratology. In Wilson JG , Fraser FC (eds): *Handbook of Teratology.* New York: Plenum, 1977, pp 47–74.
7. Kline J, Stein ZA, Susser M, Warburton D: Smoking: A risk factor for spontaneous abortion. *New England Journal of Medicine* 1977, 297:793–796.
8. Alberman E, Creasy M, Elliott M, Spicer C: Maternal factors associated with fetal chromosomal anomalies in spontaneous abortions. *British Journal of Obstetrics and Gynaecology* 1976, 83:621–627.
9. Slotkin TA, Orband-Miller L, Queen KL, Whitmore WL, Seidler FJ: Effects of prenatal nicotine exposure on biochemical development of rat brain regions: Maternal drug infusions via osmotic minipumps. *Journal of Pharmacology and Experimental Therapeutics* 1987, 240:602–611.
10. Daeninck PJ, Messiha N, Persaud TV: Intrauterine development in the rat following continuous exposure to nicotine from gestational day 6 through 12. *Anatomischer Anzeiger* 1991, 172:257–261.
11. Dobbing J: Vulnerable periods in brain growth and somatic growth. In Roberts DF, Thomson AM (eds): *The Biology of Human Fetal Growth, Volume 15, Symposia of the Society for the Study of Human Biology.* London: Taylor and Francis, 1976, pp 137–147.

12. Cairns NJ, Wonnacott S: [^{3}H](-)nicotine binding sites in fetal human brain. *Brain Research* 1988, 475:1–7.
13. Kinney HC, O'Donnell TJ, Kriger P, White WF: Early developmental changes in the [^{3}H]nicotine binding sites in the human brainstem. *Neuroscience* 1993, 55:1127–1138.
14. Kramer MS: Determinants of low birth weight; methodological assessment and meta-analysis. Bulletin of the World Health Organization 1987, 65:663–737.
15. Haddow JE, Knight GJ, Palomaki GE, Kloza EM, Wald NJ: Cigarette consumption and serum cotinine in relation to birthweight. *British Journal of Obstetrics and Gynaecology* 1987, 94:678–681.
16. Haworth JC, Ford JD: Comparison of the effects of maternal undernutrition and exposure to cigarette smoke of the cellular growth of the rat fetus. *American Journal of Obstetrics and Gynecology* 1972, 112:653–656.
17. MacArthur C, Knox EG: Smoking in pregnancy: Effects of stopping at different stages. *British Journal of Obstetrics and Gynaecology* 1988, 95:551–555.
18. Butler NR, Goldstein H: Smoking in pregnancy and subsequent child development. *British Medical Journal* 1973, 4:573–575.
19. Miller HC, Hassanein K, Hensleigh PA: Fetal growth retardation in relation to maternal smoking and weight gain in pregnancy. *American Journal of Obstetrics and Gynecology* 1976, 125:55–60.
20. Johns JM, Louis TM, Becker RF, Means LW: Behavioral effects of prenatal exposure to nicotine in guinea pigs. *Neurobehavioral Toxicology Teratology* 1982, 4:365–369.
21. Rowell PP, Sastry BV: The influence of cholinergic blockade on the uptake of alpha-aminoisobutryric acid by isolated human placental villi. *Toxicology and Applied Pharmacology* 1978, 45:79–93.
22. Wilkening RB: The role of uterine blood flow in fetal oxygen and nutrient delivery. Rosenfeld CR (ed): *The Uterine Circulation.* Ithaca: Perinatology Press, 1989, pp 191–205.
23. Greiss FC: Uterine blood flow: An overview since Barcroft. Rosenfeld CR (ed): *The Uterine Circulation.* Ithaca: Perinatology Press, 1989, pp 3–15.
24. Ford SP: Factors controlling uterine blood flow during estrous and early pregnancy. Rosenfeld CR (ed): *The Uterine Circulation.* Ithaca: Perinatology Press, 1989, pp 113–129.
25. Philipp K, Pateisky N, Endler M: Effects of smoking on uteroplacental blood flow. *Gynecologic and Obstetric Investigation* 1984, 17:179–182.
26. Lehtovirta P, Forss M: The acute effect of smoking on intervillous blood flow of the placenta. *British Journal of Obstetrics and Gynaecology* 1978, 85:729–731.
27. Mochizuki M, Maruo T, Masuko K, Ohtsu T: Effects of smoking on the fetoplacental–maternal system during pregnancy. *American Journal of Obstetrics and Gynecology* 1984, 149:413–420.
28. Naeye RL: Effects of maternal cigarette smoking on the fetus and placenta. *British Journal of Obstetrics and Gynaecology* 1978, 85:732–737.
29. Clark KE, Irion GL: Fetal hemodynamic response to maternal intravenous nicotine administration. *American Journal of Obstetrics and Gynecology* 1992, 167:1624–1631.
30. Castro LC, Allen R, Ogunyemi D, Roll K, Platt LD: Cigarette smoking during pregnancy: Acute effects on uterine flow velocity waveforms. *Obstetrics and Gynecology* 1993, 81:551–555.
31. Morrow RJ, Knox Ritchie JW, Bull SB: Maternal cigarette smoking: The effects on uterine and umbilical blood flow velocity. *American Journal of Obstetrics and Gynecology* 1988, 159:1069–1071.

32. Lindblad A, Marsal K, Andersson KE: Effect of nicotine on human fetal blood flow. *Obstetrics and Gynecology* 1988, 72:371–382.

33. Kelly J, Mathews KA, O'Conor M: Smoking in pregnancy: effects on mother and fetus. *British Journal of Obstetrics and Gynaecology* 1984, 91:111–117.

34. Resnik R, Brink GW, Wilkes M: Catecholamine mediated reduction in uterine blood flow after nicotine infusion in the pregnant ewe. *Journal of Clinical Investigation* 1979, 63:1133–1136.

35. Suzuki K, Horiguchi T, Comas-Urratia AC, Mueller-Heubach E, Adamsons K: Pharmacologic effects of nicotine upon the fetus and mother in the rhesus monkey. *American Journal of Obstetrics and Gynecology* 1971, 111:1092–1101.

36. Resnik R, Conover WB, Key TC, VanVunakis H: Uterine blood flow and catecholamine response to repetitive nicotine exposure in the pregnant ewe. *American Journal of Obstetrics and Gynecology* 1985, 151:885–891.

37. Quigley ME, Sheehan KL, Wilkes MM, Yen SS: Effects of maternal smoking on circulating catecholamine levels and fetal heart rates. *American Journal of Obstetrics and Gynecology* 1979, 133:685–690.

38. Benowitz NL, Fitzgerald GA, Wilson M, Zhang QI: Nicotine effects on eicosanoid formation and hemostatic function: Comparison of transdermal nicotine and cigarette smoking. *Journal of the American College of Cardiology* 1993, 22:1159–1167.

39. Lehtovirta P, Forss M, Rauramo I, Kariniemi V: Acute effects of nicotine on fetal heart rate variability. *British Journal of Obstetrics and Gynaecology* 1983, 90:710–715.

40. Bruner JP, Forouzan I: Smoking and buccally administered nicotine: Acute effects of uterine and umbilical artery Doppler flow velocity waveforms. *Journal of Reproductive Medicine* 1991, 36:435–440.

41. Milart P, Kauffels W, Schneider J: Vasoactive effects of nicotine in human umbilical arteries. *Zentralblatt fur Gynakologie* 1994, 116:217–219.

42. Arbeille P, Bosc M, Vaillant MC, Tranquart F: Nicotine-induced changes in the cerebral circulation in ovine fetuses. *American Journal of Perinatology* 1992, 9:270–274.

43. Manning FA, Walker D, Feyerabend C: The effect of nicotine on fetal breathing movements in conscious pregnant ewes. *Obstetrics and Gynecology* 1978, 52:563–68.

44. Manning FA, Feyerabend C: Cigarette smoking and fetal breathing movements. *British Journal of Obstetrics and Gynaecology* 1976, 83:262–270.

45. Gennser G, Marsal K, Brantmark B: Maternal smoking and fetal breathing movements. *American Journal of Obstetrics and Gynecology* 1975, 123:861–867.

46. Fitzgerald GA, Oates JA, Nowak J: Cigarette smoking and hemostatic function. *American Heart Journal* 1988, 115:267–271.

47. Marcoux S, Brisson J, Fabia J: The effect of cigarette smoking on the risk of preeclampsia and gestational hypertension. *American Journal of Epidemiology* 1989, 130:950–957.

48. Ahlsten G, Ewald U, Tuvemo T: Prostacyclin-like activity in umbilical arteries is dose-dependently reduced by maternal smoking and related to nicotine levels. *Biology of the Neonate* 1990, 58:271–278.

49. Oncken CA, Hatsukami DK, Lupo VR, Lando HA, Gibeau LM, Hansen RJ: Effects of short-term use of nicotine gum in pregnant smokers. *Clinical Pharmacology and Therapeutics.* 1996, 59:654–661.

Behavioral Toxicity of Nicotine

Nicotine is psychoactive and causes the addiction that sustains tobacco use. The psychoactive effects of nicotine are of concern in the use of nicotine as a medication.

Various aspects of the behavioral toxicity of nicotine are reviewed in Part IV. The abuse liability of nicotine as a medication is examined. Methods of testing abuse liability and the importance of pharmacokinetic factors in determining abuse liability are described. The potential toxicity of nicotine related to the development of physical dependence and/or intoxication is also reviewed. Finally, data on the risk of developing dependence on nicotine administered as a medication in various clinical trials are summarized. The findings reported in Part IV are useful in understanding the potential behavioral toxicity of various nicotine medications and in designing safety studies of newly developed nicotine medications.

Chapter 12

Abuse Liability of Nicotine

MAXINE L. STITZER and HARRIET DE WIT

Abuse liability is one aspect of a drug's pharmacology that must be considered in evaluating toxicity. It is usually regarded as an undesirable property of drugs, leading to dependence and associated physical and behavioral hazards. If a compound is found to have high abuse liability, measures to restrict access by the general population may be required. Restricted access may thus be needed even in the case of medically useful compounds such as nicotine replacement products, developed for use as smoking cessation aids. This chapter outlines the definitions and methods used to assess abuse liability of drugs; establishes some of the pharmacokinetic factors that influence abuse liability of drugs in general and nicotine in particular; and examines the comparative abuse liabilities of new nicotine delivery products, including nasal spray and vapor inhaler aerosol.

Definition and measurement of abuse liability

The likelihood that a drug will be self-administered, including the frequency and chronicity of its use, constitutes the first and most valid criterion for abuse liability. When this criterion alone is applied, the assessment might more accurately be called "use liability." Self-administration studies are most often conducted with laboratory animals such as rats and monkeys. Animals will self-administer nicotine by the intravenous route, although the behavior occurs under a more limited set of circumstances than is the case with other drugs of abuse.[1,2] Notably, however, there are no animal models currently available for self-administration of drugs either by the inhaled route or by other novel routes (e.g., buccal, nasal) that are used for delivery of nicotine in humans. Thus, animal self-administration models have limited utility at present for understanding the abuse liabilities of new nicotine delivery systems. In the case of humans, self-administration of nicotine when delivered in tobacco cigarettes is well established.

A second factor that must be taken into account when assessing abuse liability is the extent to which adverse consequences are associated with use of the drug. These adverse consequences may include acute intoxication and performance impairment as well as long-term medical consequences of chronic use. Thus, a drug such as caffeine that is regularly self-administered without significant adverse consequences may be judged to lack abuse liability. In the case of cigarettes, the adverse long-term health consequences are clearly established.[3,4] Both the acute effects and the long-term health consequences of formulations that deliver pure nicotine remain to be established. In the case of nicotine delivery systems that are used as smoking cessation aids, any adverse consequences identified must also be balanced against therapeutic benefits from tobacco smoking cessation. Finally, it should be noted that the presence of some abuse liability may actually be of benefit for a therapeutic medication. For example, a therapeutic medication that produces pleasant subjective effects may support better treatment compliance with a consequent beneficial effect on treatment outcome.

While patterns and consequences of use in the natural environment are the ultimate source of data for abuse liability, it is also important to have testing methods that can identify abuse liability prior to marketing of new products. In this regard, subjective or mood-altering effects of drugs in humans are considered to be one of the most important and reliable indices of abuse liability,[5-7] and subjective effects testing is extensively used for premarketing surveillance of new compounds. The methodology of abuse liability assessment is relatively straightforward and based on procedures developed and perfected at the National Institute on Drug Abuse (NIDA) Addiction Research Center.[8]

Experienced users of the class of drugs most closely related to the compound under assessment are typically brought into a controlled laboratory situation where they are given, on separate, independent occasions, doses of the test compound and doses of relevant comparison drugs. Following administration, they are asked to rate their subjective experiences on a variety of questions. These questions frequently include general evaluation of drug strength, as well as ratings of specific drug-produced effects associated with the class of drug being tested (stimulant, sedative, opioid). In addition, subjects are asked to rate the extent to which the drug makes them feel intoxicated or "high" and the extent to which they like or enjoy the current test drug. These ratings constitute a core element of abuse liability testing, as they indicate the judgment of experienced users concerning the desirability of the test compound.

Abuse liability comparisons

When one attempts to assess abuse liability, it is important to remember that for a particular substance this is a relative matter and must be considered in relation to other appropriate comparison compounds. In the case of a new therapeutic product, for example, one relevant comparison is with other similar therapeutic products. For example, in evaluating nicotine nasal spray and vapor inhaler, it would be relevant to compare these with other existing therapeutic products including gum and patch. Cigarettes are also a highly relevant comparison in the case of nicotine, since this is the nicotine delivery product with highest known abuse liability. It is also relevant to compare the abuse liability of nicotine with that of other drugs of abuse such as cocaine. This comparison is particularly relevant for decisions relating to control of new medications. Note that this comparison is made under controlled laboratory testing conditions, where extraneous features of the drug-taking environment are equated for the two substances. Thus, abuse liability testing provides an unbiased assessment of subjective effects that can be used to predict use in the natural environment. This controlled testing does not take into account other important factors such as availability, social acceptability, and product promotion, which can also clearly exert an important influence on prevalence of use in the natural environment.

Pharmacokinetic factors in abuse liability

In assessing the abuse liability of drugs, it is important to consider the pharmacokinetics of drug delivery. Pharmacokinetic factors are particularly important to understand in evaluating the abuse liability of nicotine because this drug is delivered in several different formulations that result in markedly different pharmacokinetic profiles.

Speed of drug effects onset

The first important factor is the speed of onset of the drug effect. This includes both the latency to initial perception of a drug's subjective effects and the rate of increase of the drug's subjective effects, or the time from the first perceptible effect to the peak effect. The importance of plasma rise time and consequent rate of drug effect onset is illustrated by two studies conducted with human subjects in which this feature of drug delivery was experimentally manipulated.[9,10] Both studies addressed the question of whether the rate of change of blood levels would influence the pleasant or euphorigenic subjective effects of the drug; the test compound employed was either pentobarbital[9] or diazepam.[10] In both studies, drug was administered as a single bolus in one experimental condition, while in a second condition the drug was administered in divided doses over a 2-hour period. The dose magnitude was adjusted to achieve equivalent peak plasma levels. These different methods of administration produced different rise time, but equivalent peak plasma concentrations, as expected. In both studies, subjects could distinguish active drug from placebo. However, when the drug was delivered under the bolus dose rapid onset condition, it was rated as more intoxicating and euphorigenic than when administered under the divided dose condition. This is illustrated for pentobarbital in Figure 12-1. These controlled studies illustrate that plasma rise time and consequent rate of drug effect onset play an important role in abuse liability, independent of peak plasma levels.

With nicotine, the route of administration has an important influence on the pharmacokinetic profile of the drug. Figure 12-2 illustrates plasma venous nicotine concentrations achieved after subjects smoked a single cigarette (10 puffs in 6 minutes), administered a 2-mg dose of nasal gel (precursor to the recently marketed nasal spray), chewed a 2-mg piece of nicotine polacrilex gum for 30 minutes[11] or puffed to maximum exertion for 20 minutes using Favor, a previously test-marketed smoke-free cigarette that delivers a unit dose of 0.013 mg of nicotine per puff.[12] These administration regimens represent doses at or above the therapeutic range (2 mg of nasal spray is twice the recommended acute therapeutic dose; pharmacokinetic data for the 1-mg nasal spray are presented in an article by Schneider et al.[13] It is clear that the plasma profiles are similar for nicotine delivered via absorption through the lungs (cigarettes) and through the nasal mucosa in that both exhibit rapid increase in nicotine levels. In contrast, plasma levels rise much more gradually for gum and vapor inhaler. Nicotine absorption with the gum is limited by mechanics of the gradual release of nicotine from the polacrilex resin. The slow rise time for vapor inhaler suggests that absorption is primarily through membranes of the mouth and upper airway rather than lung alveoli. This slow rise time also reflects the effort necessary to administer significant doses with a device that delivers a very small unit puff dose. Nicotine patch has an even slower plasma rise time, on the order of hours rather than minutes.[14,15] These observations suggest that nicotine delivery systems would differ with regard to the intensity of subjective effects produced, with most intense effects produced by cigarettes followed by nasal spray, vapor inhaler, gum, and, finally, patch. A 1995 study by Wakasa et al.[16] confirmed in an animal self-administration model that plasma rise time influences the reinforcing properties of nicotine. Rhesus monkeys self-administered nicotine intravenously for 24 hours per day under a fixed ratio 5 schedule of lever pressing with a 15 minute time out after each drug injection. The investigators experimentally manipulated infusion speed (from 5.2 to 0.3 µg /sec) of a fixed (30 µg/kg per infusion) unit dose of nicotine. They observed that the monkeys self-administered more nicotine in 24 hours under the faster than the slower infusion speed conditions.

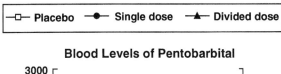

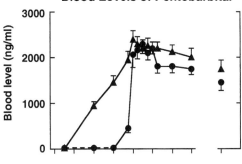

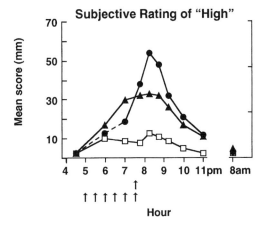

Figure 12-1. Blood levels of pentobarbital; subjective rating of "high." Top: Blood levels of pentobarbital are shown as a function of clock hours during and after administration of a 180-mg oral divided dose given as six 30-mg doses at 30-minute intervals (closed triangles) and after a single bolus 150-mg oral dose of pentobarbital (closed circles). In both cases, subjects ingested six capsules under double-blind conditions; in the bolus dose condition, five of these contained placebo. In a third condition (not shown), all capsules contained placebo. Active dose administrations are indicated by vertical arrows shown under the abscissa (i.e., single bolus dose administered at 7:30 p.m.). Means represent data from 12 human subjects; brackets are ± SEM. Bottom: Subjective ratings on the question "Are you high?" "Subjects made a vertical mark along a 100-mm line labeled "none"/"not at all" at one end and "a lot"/"very much" at the other, according to how they felt at that moment. Means are shown for 12 subjects who received placebo, sodium pentobarbital (150 mg) in a single bolus dose, or sodium pentobarbital (180 mg total) in six divided doses spaced at 30-minute intervals. Conditions were tested in counterbalanced order across three experimental sessions. (Data from de Wit et al.[9])

123

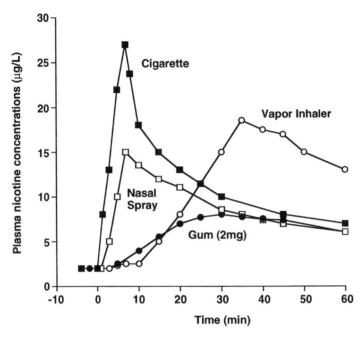

Figure 12-2. Plasma nicotine concentrations during and after drug administration are shown for four different nicotine delivery systems. The cigarette had standard machine-smoked deliveries of 17 mg tar and 1.4 mg nicotine, but was expected to deliver about 2 mg nicotine under controlled puffing conditions. Subjects were instructed to inhale one puff as deeply as possible every 40 seconds for a total of 10 puffs in 6 minutes. Nasal nicotine was administered at time 0 in a single dose containing 2 mg nicotine at pH 5.0 without added buffer; viscosity of the fluid was increased with a cellulose derivative. Nicotine chewing gum was the commercially available product containing 2 mg nicotine and was chewed for 30 minutes. Data for cigarettes, nasal spray, and gum are means of three subjects. Vapor inhaler data were obtained using Favor cigarettes, which nominally delivered 13 µg per 50 mg puff at 21° Celsius. The first test cigarette was puffed at intervals of 40 seconds to a total of 10 puffs in 6 minutes. After a 4-minute pause, there followed a period of maximal puffing in which the subjects puffed and inhaled as hard and as frequently as possible for 20 minutes, changing every 5 minutes to a fresh cigarette. Vapor inhaler data are a mean of eight subjects. (Modified from Schneider NG: Nicotine Therapy in Smoking Cessation. Pharmacokinetic Considerations. *Clinical Pharmacokinetics* 1992, 23:169–172.)

Peak effect magnitude

The second pharmacokinetic factor that should be taken into account is the magnitude of the peak plasma level. With most drugs of abuse, higher peak blood concentrations entail higher risk for abuse. Thus, higher doses of a given drug, which produce higher blood concentrations, are generally chosen over lower doses, indicating their greater abuse liability.[17] Other things being equal, a formulation or a route of administration that leads to a lower peak level would generally be associated with lower abuse potential. In Figure 12-2, the cigarette produced the highest peak level of nicotine, nasal gel and vapor inhaler produced an intermediate peak level, and the nicotine gum an even lower peak level. The differential between cigarette and nasal peak plasma levels occurred despite the nasal gel delivering twice the recommended therapeutic dose. However, because patients control their own doses of products using various delivery routes, the data suggest that it might be possible to take a higher dose of a nasal product and achieve pharmacokinetics and peak levels similar to those produced by cigarettes. Likewise, higher peak levels could be achieved with gum by using a more potent formulation, and higher levels are theoretically possible with vapor inhaler by making a product that delivers a larger dose per puff.

Arterial/venous plasma ratio

Another pharmacokinetic factor that is relevant, particularly for an inhaled drug such as nicotine, is the ratio of the arterial levels to the venous levels of drug following administration. Henningfield and colleagues[18] have demonstrated that there can be up to a 10-fold higher concentration of drug in the arterial blood than in the venous blood immediately after smoking a cigarette. Nicotine is absorbed from the lung alveoli into the arterial system and travels directly to the brain, where it delivers high concentrations of the drug at central sites of action. Nicotine may reach the brain within 10–20 seconds after smoke inhalation. This rapid delivery of a high dose to central nervous system sites makes the inhalation route a particularly pernicious one in terms of abuse liability. No other currently known nicotine delivery product uses this route of administration; nasal spray is thought to be primarily absorbed in the nasal mucosa, and vapor inhaler appears to deliver nicotine primarily to the upper airways rather than the alveoli. This suggests that both systems would deliver nicotine more slowly to the arterial circulation than cigarette smoking would. If true, this would suggest that both nasal spray and vapor inhaler would have lower abuse liability than cigarettes based on these blood distribution patterns. However, confirmation is needed for these assertions with empirical data on arterial to venous ratios produced by other nicotine delivery products.

Plasma half-life

The duration of effect associated with drug half-life in the body is another pharmacokinetic factor that may influence liability for abuse, and it may do so by determining the frequency of drug self-administration. Specifically, a longer duration of effect might result in less frequent administrations and fewer repeated exposures within a given time frame. Nicotine has a very short half-life of approximately 2 hours,[19] resulting in the need for frequent self-administration. However, slow, steady absorption, such as that achieved with transdermal patch, would be less likely to support frequent use, other things being equal.

Pharmacokinetic implications

Overall, the data show that pharmacokinetic properties of drug delivery vary greatly with different delivery systems and that plasma level profiles can have a strong influence on abuse liability of drugs. With regard to the new nicotine delivery systems, the plasma profile of nicotine delivered via a nasal system appears to be more similar to that observed with cigarette smoking than with use of polacrilex gum, while nicotine delivered in a vapor inhaler has a slower plasma rise time, more similar to that seen with gum. The data further suggest that it may be possible to rank the relative abuse liabilities of nicotine delivery products based on their pharmacokinetic properties. Specifically, the data suggest that cigarettes would have the highest abuse liability because of rapid onset of effects, high peak plasma levels, and high arterial/venous concentrations. Nasal spray would have the next highest abuse liability, since this system also achieves rapid plasma rise time. Vapor inhaler and gum would follow with slower rise times and lower peak concentrations. The patch, which requires several hours to reach peak levels, would have the lowest abuse liability. These predictions from pharmacokinetic data could be modified by other factors and must be verified through direct testing of subjective effects and self-administration behavior.

Subjective effects assessment of nicotine abuse liability

In contrast to other drugs of abuse, nicotine produces relatively little actual subjective intoxication or experience of "high." Moreover, its direct subjective effects are somewhat elusive and difficult to characterize. It is clear, however, that human subjects can, under appropriate circumstances, identify the presence of nicotine and report subjective experiences that result from its administration. Subjective effects are also influenced by the delivery system used to administer nicotine.

"Liking" ratings

The top two panels of Figure 12-3 present data generated by Henningfield and colleagues[20] from a study in which nicotine was either inhaled in cigarette smoke or received intravenously by subjects who were both cigarette smokers and drug abusers. Subjects detected the presence of a drug and indicated that they liked the drug effects; in both cases, subjective report scores were dose related—the larger the dose, the more "liking" was reported. Data collected for nicotine nasal spray and vapor inhaler,[21] gum,[22] and patch,[23] which are presented in the remaining panels of Figure 12-3, stand in contrast to the data for inhaled and intravenous nicotine. When the drug was administered in these alternative dosing forms, across a range of doses, subjects did not report any "liking."

"Good" and "bad" effect ratings

The "liking" question provides a composite assessment of pleasant and unpleasant subjective effects. Thus, it is worthwhile to examine subjective reports in more detail by asking questions that specifically tap these opposing dimensions. A laboratory test of acute subjective effects of cigarettes, nasal spray, and vapor inhaler was conducted at the Behavioral Pharmacology Research Unit, Johns Hopkins, in collaboration with the National Institutes of Health, NIDA, Addiction Research Center.[21]

The subjects were 12 regular smokers who received acute doses of nasal spray (0, 1, 2, and 4 sprays, each delivering 0.5 mg nicotine); vapor inhaler (0, 30, 60, and 120 puffs, each delivering 0.13 mg nicotine); and cigarettes (0, 4, 8, and 16 puffs, from a cigarette with a rated yield of 1 mg nicotine) under double-blind conditions. In this study, "liking" scores were elevated after subjects smoked cigarettes, but not after administration of nasal spray or vapor inhaler (see Fig. 12-3). However, scores on a "good drug effects" rating increased following both nasal spray and vapor inhaler. Although the magnitude of the increase on the "good effects" rating was greater after cigarettes than after either of the novel delivery systems, the data nevertheless suggest that these delivery systems are not without some abuse liability. Subject ratings of "bad drug effects" increased markedly after nasal spray and vapor inhaler, but not after cigarettes. No specific side effects were reported for cigarettes. In contrast, a plethora of unpleasant side effects were reported after nasal spray, including throat irritation, coughing, burning nose, runny nose, sneezing, and watery eyes. Vapor inhaler was associated with throat irritation and coughing. These reported side effects are consistent with findings from previous clinical studies in which these nicotine delivery systems were tested.[24]

Implications of abuse liability testing

The profile of effects obtained during this acute testing protocol suggests that the potential abuse liability of both nasal spray and vapor inhaler is lower than that of cigarettes. Based on the pharmacokinetic profile alone, nasal spray would be expected to have abuse liability similar to that of cigarettes because of fast plasma rise time. However, data from clinical trials[24,25] and from the laboratory abuse liability study described above suggest that abuse liability of nasal spray and vapor inhaler is modulated by unpleasant side effects. Unpleasant side effects might limit both acceptability of these new products and compliance with their use by

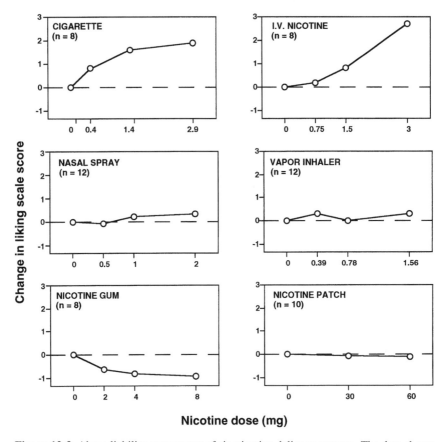

Nicotine dose (mg)

Figure 12-3. Abuse liability assessment of six nicotine delivery systems. The data shown are ratings on scales measuring subjective drug liking. In each case, liking scores after placebo administration were subtracted from liking scores obtained after active dose administration. Except for patch, the data shown were obtained immediately after active dose administration. For cigarettes and intravenous nicotine, subjects rated drug liking on a scale of 0 = "not at all" to 4 = "awful lot" following acute test doses. Subjects were smokers with histories of drug abuse. Cigarettes were obtained from the Tobacco and Health Research Institute of Kentucky and had machine-rated nicotine deliveries of 0.4, 1.4, and 2.9 mg nicotine when tested using the same smoking conditions employed in the study (1-second puffs at 30-second intervals until a 23-mm butt length was reached); 0 mg = sham smoking. Intravenous nicotine was administered as 10-second infusions; doses are as nicotine base. For nasal spray and vapor inhaler, subjects rated "How much do you like the medication?" along a 100-mm analog scale with 0 = "not at all" to 100 = "extremely." Scores were converted to a 0 to 4 scale for this presentation. Subjects were regular smokers without histories of drug abuse. During testing of nasal spray and vapor inhaler, subjects always took a fixed number of sprays (4) or aerosol inhalations (120), with the number of administrations that contained active versus placebo drug varied according to test condition and active doses presented at the end of the administration period. The active nasal product delivered 0.5 mg nicotine per spray; the active inhaler delivered 0.013 mg nicotine per inhalation. For gum, liking was rated on a scale from 0 = "not at all" to 4 = "an awful lot." Subjects, regular smokers without histories of drug abuse, chewed two pieces

tobacco-dependent patients in treatment. The side effects might also limit initial use and abuse of these products by nicotine-naive individuals (i.e., nonsmokers). It should be noted, however, that cigarettes also have unpleasant side effects in naive users, and this does not seem to act as a major deterrent to initiation of use. Furthermore, with regard to regular smokers, it is clear from clinical trials that smokers who are motivated to quit can grow accustomed to the side effects of nasal spray and vapor inhaler over time and may even report positive subjective effects (other than withdrawal relief) from their use.[24,26,27] For example, in one study by Sutherland and colleagues,[24] 56% of active spray subjects compared with 39% of those using placebo spray reported good or "high" feelings from use of nasal spray at least once during the first month of treatment ($p < 0.05$). Similarly, in a study by Hajek and colleagues[28] that employed a smoke-free cigarette similar to the current vapor inhaler, satisfaction ratings during a 24-hour period of smoking abstinence were twice as high when active than when placebo nicotine delivery devices were used. An additional abuse liability study testing acute effects in individuals habituated to the use of these nicotine delivery systems would be informative. Nevertheless, the subjective report data, overall, support the assertion that nasal spray and vapor inhaler, while not completely devoid of abuse liability, have abuse liabilities lower than that of cigarettes.

Conclusions

Nicotine clearly has abuse liability, as exemplified by its role in cigarette smoking. However, and perhaps to a greater extent than other drugs of abuse, nicotine's abuse liability is modulated by route of administration and resulting pharmacokinetic profiles as well as other characteristics of the delivery system.

Nicotine inhaled via cigarettes lies at the high end of an abuse liability continuum. Inhaled nicotine is associated with rapid plasma rise time, high peak plasma levels, and a high arterial/venous ratio. These characteristics result in rapid onset of effects and delivery of high bolus doses directly to the brain. At the other end of the continuum is the nicotine patch, with extremely long plasma rise times in the range of hours rather than minutes. Nicotine gum, nasal spray, and vapor aerosols, new delivery products designed as cessation aids, fall somewhere along this continuum of abuse liability depending on a composite set of factors including plasma rise times, side effect profiles, and effort needed to obtain significant doses.

---

of gum simultaneously for 20 minutes with one chew every 3 seconds. For patch, liking ratings were obtained during chronic testing of three patch doses; subjects were exposed to each patch dose for 1 week. Subjects were smokers; half did and half did not have histories of drug abuse. (Data from Henningfield et al.,[20] Schuh et al.,[21] Nemeth-Coslett et al.,[22] and Bunker et al.[23])

Overall, the data support the conclusion that cigarettes remain the most highly abusable nicotine delivery product. Given this observation, the purposeful abuse of new nicotine delivery products either by current smokers or new initiates seems unlikely as long as cigarettes are available on a cost-competitive basis. When considering the role of abuse liability in medications development, it is important to remember that some pleasurable subjective effects might be desirable because medications with such effects may support better treatment compliance and improved clinical outcomes.

Acknowledgments

Preparation of this chapter was supported, in part, by USPHS/NIH grant DA03893 from the National Institute on Drug Abuse, National Institutes of Health.

References

1. Corrigall WA, Cohen KM: Nicotine maintains robust self-administration in rats on a limited-access schedule. *Brain Research* 1989, 99:473–478.
2. Tessari M, Valerio E, Chiamulera C, Beardsley PM: Nicotine reinforcement in rats with histories of cocaine self-administration. *Psychopharmacology* 1995, 121:282–283.
3. U.S. Department of Health, Education and Welfare, Public Health Service, Office of the Assistant Secretary for Health, Office on Smoking and Health: *A Report of the Surgeon General.* Washington, DC: Department of Health, Education and Welfare, Publication 79–50066, 1979.
4. U.S. Department of Health and Human Services, Public Health Service, Centers for Disease Control, Center on Smoking and Health: *Reducing the Health Consequences of Smoking: 25 Years of Progress.* A Report of the Surgeon General. Washington, DC: Department of Health and Human Services, Publication 89–8411, 1989.
5. Fischman MW, Foltin RW: Utility of subjective-effects measurements in assessing abuse liability of drugs in humans. *British Journal of Addiction* 1991, 86:1563–1570.
6. Foltin RW, Fischman MW: Methods for the assessment of abuse liability of psychomotor stimulants and anorectic agents in humans. *British Journal of Addiction* 1991, 86:1633–1640.
7. Jasinski DR: History of abuse liability testing in humans. *British Journal of Addiction* 1991, 86:1559–1562.
8. Jasinski DR: Assessment of the abuse potentiality of morphine-like drug (methods used in man). In Martin WR (ed): *Handbook of Experimental Pharmacology Vol 45: Drug Addiction I,* Heidelberg: Springer-Verlag. 1977, pp 197–258.
9. de Wit H, Bodker B, Ambre J: Rate of increase of plasma drug influences subjective response in humans. *Psychopharmacology* 1992, 107:352–358.
10. de Wit H, Dudish S, Ambre J: Subjective and behavioral effects of diazepam depend on its rate of onset. *Psychopharmacology* 1993, 112:324–330.
11. Russell MAH, Jarvis MJ, Feyerabend C, Ferno O: Nasal nicotine solution: a potential aid to giving up smoking? *British Medical Journal* 1983, 286:683–684.
12. Russell MAH, Jarvis MJ, Sutherland G, Feyerabend C: Nicotine replacement in smoking cessation. Absorption of nicotine vapor from smoke-free cigarettes. *Journal of the American Medical Association* 1987, 257:3262–3265.
13. Schneider NG, Lunell E, Olmstead RE, Fagerstrom K: Clinical pharmacokinetics of

nasal nicotine delivery. A review and comparison to other nicotine systems. *Clinical Pharmacokinetics* 1996, 31:65–80.

14. Benowitz NL, Chan K, Denaro CP, Jacob P: Stable isotope method for studying transdermal drug absorption: The nicotine patch. *Clinical Pharmacology and Therapeutics* 1991, 50:286–293.

15. Gorsline J, Gupta SK, Dye D, Rolf CN: Steady-state pharmacokinetics and dose relationship of nicotine delivered from Nicoderm (nicotine transdermal system). *Journal of Clinical Pharmacology* 1993, 33:161–168.

16. Wakasa Y, Takada K, Yanagita T: Reinforcing effect as a function of infusion speed in intravenous self-administration of nicotine in rhesus monkeys. *Japanese Journal of Psychopharmacology* 1995, 15:53–59.

17. Johanson CE, Schuster CR: Animal models of drug self-administration. In Mello NK (ed): *Advances in Substance Abuse 2.* Greenwich, CT: Jai Press, 1981, pp 219–297.

18. Henningfield JE, Stapleton JM, Benowitz NL, Grayson RF, London ED: Higher levels of nicotine in arterial than in venous blood after cigarette smoking. *Drug and Alcohol Dependence* 1993, 33:23–29.

19. Benowitz NL, Jacob P, Jones RT, Rosenberg J: Interindividual variability in the metabolism and cardiovascular effects of nicotine in man. *Journal of Pharmacology and Experimental Therapeutics* 1982, 221:368–372.

20. Henningfield JE, Miyasato K, Jasinski DR: Abuse liability and pharmacodynamic characteristics of intravenous and inhaled nicotine. *Journal of Pharmacology and Experimental Therapeutics* 1985, 234:1–12.

21. Schuh KJ, Schuh LM, Henningfield JE, Stitzer ML: Nicotine nasal spray and vapor inhaler: abuse liability assessment. *Psychopharmacology* 1997, 130:352–361.

22. Nemeth-Coslett R, Henningfield JE, O'Keefe MK, Griffiths RR: Nicotine gum: Dose-related effects on cigarette smoking and subjective effects. *Psychopharmacology* 1987, 92:424–430.

23. Bunker EB, Pickworth WB, Henningfield JE: Nicotine patch: Effect on spontaneous smoking. In Harris L (ed): *Problems of Drug Dependence 1991.* National Insitutes of Health, National Institute on Drug Abuse, Research Monograph 119. Department of Health and Human Services Publication 92–1888, 1992, p 470.

24. Sutherland G, Stapleton JA, Russell MAH, Jarvis MJ, Hajek P, Belcher M, Feyerabend C: Randomized controlled trial of nasal nicotine spray in smoking cessation. *Lancet* 1992, 340:324–329.

25. Hjalmarson A, Franzon M, Westin A, Wiklund O: Effect of nicotine nasal spray on smoking cessation. *Archives of Internal Medicine* 1994, 154:2567–2572.

26. Jarvis MJ, Hajek P, Russell MAH, West RJ, Feyerabend C: Nasal nicotine solution as an aid to cigarette withdrawal: A pilot clinical trial. *British Journal of Addiction* 1987, 82:983–988.

27. Tonnesen P, Norregaard J, Mikkelsen K, Jorgensen S, Nilsson F: Double-blind trial of nicotine inhaler for smoking cessation. *Journal of the American Medical Association* 1993, 269:1268–1271.

28. Hajek P, Jarvis MJ, Belcher M, Sutherland G, Feyerabend C: Effect of smoke-free cigarettes on 24 hour cigarette withdrawal: A double-blind placebo-controlled study. *Psychopharmacology* 1989, 97:99–102.

Chapter 13

Behavioral Toxicology
of Nicotine

JACK E. HENNINGFIELD and STEPHEN J. HEISHMAN

Psychoactive drug use can adversely affect the physical health of the user directly and can also lead to increased morbidity and mortality because of adverse behavioral effects on users. For example, alcohol use may produce cirrhosis of the liver, and an alcohol-intoxicated automobile driver can cause an accident leading to the death of the driver or other persons.[1] Generally, marijuana use is not directly lethal to users; however, regular use leads to lung disease and other forms of toxicity,[2] and the adverse effects of marijuana on driving abilities have been documented.[3,4] Opioids may cause death due to overdose, but the more common causes of morbidity among opioid users are the side effects resulting from the dependence process, such as the development of diseases like aquired immunodeficiency syndrome and hepatitis resulting from use of contaminated drug delivery systems and impure drug.[5]

Nicotine has the potential to produce adverse physiological effects, which are discussed in other chapters in this volume. However, most of the morbidity and mortality caused by tobacco use may be considered side effects of the nicotine dependence process in that toxicity results from repeated exposure to the highly contaminated tobacco delivery systems used in an addictive manner by the vast majority of tobacco users.[6] The incidence and prevalence rates of nicotine addiction are related to the nicotine dosage form as well as to factors such as cost, availability, and social variables[7-9] (see also Chapter 12). For example, cigarettes are the most toxic and addictive form of nicotine delivery because they permit rapid delivery of controllable doses of nicotine along with sensory stimuli designed to be maximally palatable; their design both requires and reinforces inhalation of highly toxic smoke into the lung, and cigarettes are among the most readily available and highly advertised of all consumer products.[11] In contrast, nicotine transdermal patches provide relatively slow release of nicotine, no moment to moment control over dosage, and no pleasurable sensory effects and have much greater marketing and advertising restrictions[7,9] (see also Chapter 12). These factors contribute to the remarkable record of safety and low potential for abuse and dependence of transdermal patch systems.

Between the extremes of the cigarette and the nicotine transdermal patch, with respect to safety and addiction potential, are a broad range of other nicotine delivery systems that have been marketed or have the potential to be marketed by tobacco and pharmaceutical companies. These products vary in their toxic and addictive effects ,as has been discussed elsewhere[10,11] (see also Chapter 12). In principle, just as the level of addictive effects varies across nicotine delivery system, so could other adverse behavioral effects vary across nicotine delivery systems. The possibility that increasing numbers of nicotine-dependent tobacco users will achieve and sustain tobacco abstinence through protracted use of nicotine-delivering medications raises concerns about the safety and toxicity of nicotine itself and how the safety and toxicity of nicotine might be affected by the delivery system. Other chapters in this volume address the variety of potential adverse effects of nicotine on physical health. In the category of potential adverse behavioral effects, Stitzer and de Wit (Chapter 12) address the addiction potential ("abuse liability") of nicotine across different forms of nicotine delivery. The present chapter addresses other potential adverse behavioral effects of nicotine administration and withdrawal. When possible, we draw conclusions and comment on the likelihood that the nature of the nicotine delivery system would affect the severity of the effect.

Dose, speed of delivery, and tolerance influence the behavioral effects of nicotine

When attempting to predict the effects of nicotine on behavior, it is important to consider that factors in addition to the chemical structure of nicotine are relevant. In particular, it has been understood since the end of the nineteenth century that the magnitude of nicotine's effects on physiological responses is related to the dose and the degree of tolerance.[12,13] Similarly, whether a person or animal can even discriminate varying levels of administration of nicotine is directly related to the dose and inversely related to the level of tolerance.[14] Studies of the effects of speed of nicotine delivery are more limited but indicate that the kinetics of nicotine delivery are also an important determinant of effects.[7,15] For example, rapid administration of a few tenths of a milligram of nicotine in the form of cig-

arette smoke inhalation or intravenous injection can produce a significant increase in heart rate and people can discriminate the difference in level, whereas
the infusion of more than 20 mg of nicotine over 24 hours may be accompanied
by no detectable change in heart rate or ability to discriminate the drug.[15–17] The
physiological basis for the interaction between dosage and tolerance development, as well as why speed of delivery would be relevant, has been well reviewed
by Sheiner.[18] The development of tolerance to the behavioral and other effects of
nicotine has also been reviewed elsewhere.[10,13]

As discussed by Sheiner,[18] the development of tolerance to nicotine is so rapid
that slow infusions of nicotine, as provided by transdermal systems, enable the
body to develop tolerance and thus display a smaller response than would have
been predicted had the same dose been delivered more rapidly. More rapid delivery also provides larger, albeit more shortly lived, concentrations of nicotine at
nicotinic receptor sites.[15] In the extreme case, inhalation of cigarette smoke produces arterial boli, which persist only a few minutes but which may be 10 times
greater than venous concentrations.[19] A nasal nicotine delivery medication provides nicotine with sufficient rapidity to produce an approximate doubling of arterial levels relative to venous blood levels.[20] Smokeless tobacco products vary
widely in their pH[21,22] and have been shown to produce wide variation in speed of
nicotine release across a dialysis membrane model of nicotine absorption.[23,24]

Just as factors such as dose and speed of nicotine delivery are important to consider in assessing the abuse liability of a given nicotine delivery system, these
factors must also be considered in assessing other behavioral effects of nicotine.
Here it is important to keep in mind that systems vary not only in their intended
unit dosing characteristics but also in the behavioral effort required to obtain a
dose. For example, the speed of nicotine absorption from a standard dose of the
commercially marketed nicotine nasal spray appears to be only somewhat more
rapid than that provided by 4 mg of nicotine gum. However, nicotine nasal spray
enables the user to easily and quickly repeat the dosage many times during the
same period that it would take to self-administer nicotine gum. These are all factors that should be considered in predicting the behavioral effects that would be
produced by any nicotine delivery system.

Physical dependence and withdrawal influence the behavioral effects of nicotine

The repeated exposure to nicotine leads to a state of physical dependence such
that abrupt termination of nicotine administration might be accompanied by withdrawal symptoms.[10,25,26] As described in the reviews, withdrawal symptoms include disrupted performance and impaired ability to concentrate on cognitive
tasks. In fact, nicotine withdrawal symptoms were considered significant enough
by an expert panel of the U.S. Centers for Disease Control and Prevention, which

evaluated the risks of cigarette smoking by airline pilots, to conclude that "the adverse effects of withdrawal in a chronic smoker are deemed potentially significant, and may have a net adverse effect on flight safety."[27]

Withdrawal symptoms from nicotine and other drugs can be minimized by gradual reduction of dosage and by the use of replacement medications.[5,27-29] These behavioral withdrawal effects are associated with, and probably mediated by, disruptions in brain function that begin within a few hours of the last cigarette.[30]. Figure 13-1 shows data from studies that illustrate the relationship between electroencephalogram measures of brain function and behavioral performance when nicotine administration is discontinued. Figure 13-2 shows gum effects on electroencephalographic measures and behavior.

Just as the abuse liability of nicotine is substantially greater when delivered in tobacco products than when delivered in current medications[7] (see also Chapter 12), the physical dependence potential of nicotine appears to be greater when delivered via tobacco products than via current medications. For example, the symptoms of nicotine withdrawal are generally lower following nicotine medication discontinuation than following tobacco abstinence. Specifically, the most severe symptoms occur upon termination of cigarette smoking.[10,26] This is consistent with the high arterial and venous doses of nicotine produced by cigarette smoking; the rapid decline in nicotine blood levels upon termination of smoking; the plethora of oral, nasal, visual, and tactile stimuli produced by smoking cigarettes; and the ubiquitous presence of tobacco-associated stimuli in the general environment.[10] Nicotine withdrawal symptoms are qualitatively similar, but generally weaker in smokeless tobacco users than in cigarette smokers.[31] Although smokeless tobacco users can achieve similar venous nicotine blood levels as cigarette smokers, they do not obtain the arterial spikes produced by smoke inhalation, plasma levels decline more gradually,[32] and the sensory components are arguably less pronounced.

Withdrawal symptoms are generally weaker upon discontinuation of transdermal nicotine patch use than upon discontinuation of cigarettes and smokeless tobacco.[33] This is consistent with the facts that peak blood levels are generally lower with any of the patches than those typically produced by cigarette smoking and that the skin serves as a depot that continues to release nicotine for several hours after patch removal.[34,35] Although it is clear that many patients need gradual reduction of their nicotine patch dose to minimize withdrawal symptoms, it is not clear that there is a general benefit of such dose tapering in all patients.[29,33,36,37] Unfortunately, it is not possible to predict which patients would benefit from tapering a priori. It is plausible that nicotine delivery systems that enable higher levels of nicotine exposure and/or are characterized by more rapidly falling levels of nicotine following discontinuation of dosing will be accompanied by increased withdrawal symptoms after discontinuation of use.

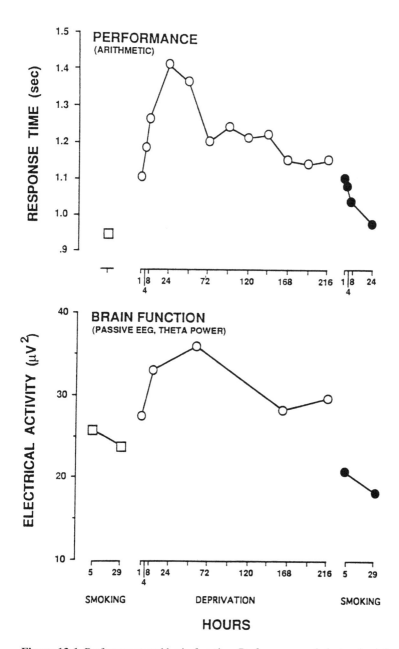

Figure 13-1. Performance and brain function. Performance and electrophysiological measures of brain function are shown in a group of volunteers while smoking (closed symbols); during 9 days of tobacco abstinence (open symbols); and after resumption of smoking. (Data from Pickworth et al.[71])

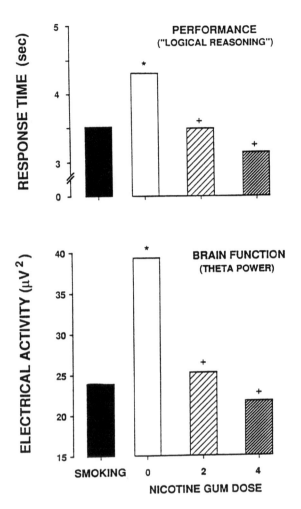

Figure 13-2. Performance and brain function: smoking and varied gum doses. Performance and an electrophysiological measure of brain function in human volunteers are shown during smoking or in the absence of tobacco after treatment with placebo or nicotine-delivery polacrilex gum. Nicotine gum or placebo was given after either 12 hours (performance study) or 29 hours (electrophysiological study) nicotine deprivation. *Significant difference from ad libitum smoking. +Significant difference from placebo gum. (Data from Pickworth et al.[71])

Effects of nicotine on behavior

Hundreds of studies have been conducted to assess the effects of nicotine on behavior, learning, and performance in animals and humans since the early twentieth century.[10,38,39] The behaviors range from simple lever-pressing tasks in animals and finger tapping in humans to complex cognitive problem solving in humans. The means of nicotine delivery include subcutaneous injections, cigarettes, cigars, nicotine gum, and nasal nicotine sprays. Many of these studies have been described in the afore-mentioned reviews and they need not be reviewed here; but, taken together, this literature supports the following conclusions:

1. Acute doses of nicotine can disrupt task performance and ongoing general behavior.[40,41]
   a. These effects generally last less than 30 minutes.
   b. The effects are most pronounced after the first exposure of the organism to the drug. Re-exposure, even months later, may produce much weaker effects.
   c. The level of behavioral tolerance is so profound that it may require doses that produce side effects such as nausea or vomiting to disrupt ongoing behavior.
2. Acute doses of nicotine can impede learning. These effects are related to the same kinds of variables as studied in research on the effects of nicotine on performance and general behavior; however, there is much less research on the effects of nicotine on complex learning than on psychomotor performance.[39]
3. In people, and possibly animals, acute doses of nicotine can restore nicotine withdrawal-associated impairment of performance and learning.[42,43]
4. Under limited conditions (e.g., motor responding), the administration of nicotine may enhance performance in individuals who are not nicotine dependent or who are dependent but not undergoing nicotine withdrawal.[39,44]
5. The magnitude of the behavioral effects is often related to the total dose, the nature of the behavioral response under study, and probably the rate of administration. However, the influence of rate must be assessed by cross-study comparisons because there is little evidence directly assessing the impact of speed of nicotine delivery on behavior.[45,46]
6. The effects of nicotine on behavior are due to the actions of nicotine on brain nicotine receptors because nicotine antagonists that act peripherally and on the central nervous system (e.g., mecamylamine) prevent the effects of nicotine, whereas nicotine antagonists that do not cross the blood–brain barrier (e.g., pentolinium or hexamethonium) have no such effect on the response to nicotine.[47,48]
7. The behavioral effects of nicotine are not accurately characterized as, generally, either stimulating or sedating because the nature of the observed effects depend on the behavior being assessed, the nicotine dose, the level of tolerance, and whether the organism appears to be in a state of nicotine withdrawal.[10]

Is nicotine an intoxicating drug?

At high doses, nicotine can severely disrupt behavior and produce intoxication.[10,13,49] Nicotine overdose or intoxication sometimes occurs in agricultural settings by people working with nicotine pesticides or those harvesting tobacco leaves.[10] It is also a frequent response to an individual's first smoking experience.[50] Interestingly, it is an effect that was apparently sought after and produced in religious and tribal ceremonies for centuries.[51] On the other hand, intoxication by nicotine is rare in regular tobacco and nicotine medication users. Therefore, the American Psychiatric Association does not list a syndrome of nicotine intoxication as a nicotine use disorder.[27] Thus, although nicotine can produce intoxication, it is not generally considered an intoxicating drug. The reasons that nicotine intoxication is rarely a phenomenon of clinical significance are summarized in an effort to illustrate how the likelihood of intoxication could be reduced or enhanced depending on the nicotine dosage form.

Nicotine intoxication is rare, primarily because of the rapidly acquired tolerance level of nicotine obtained and the fact that consumer-oriented delivery products are designed and marketed to minimize acute overdosing. For example, nicotine medications include dosing instructions in accordance with smoking level.[36,52] Smokeless tobacco products are differentially marketed according to their nicotine delivery speed capacity so that low pH (i.e., slow delivering) products are marketed more heavily to younger nonsmokeless tobacco users, and higher pH products (i.e., rapid nicotine delivering) are marketed more selectively to experienced smokeless tobacco users.[21,22,53,54] All currently marketed cigarettes appear capable of delivering sufficient nicotine to cause behavioral disruption in nontolerant people.[55] However, the advice that first-time users typically receive from experienced users and the ability to titrate nicotine on a puff-by-puff basis reduce the incidence of intoxication upon initial use.

For people who are tolerant to and dependent on tobacco products, currently available nicotine medications seem highly unlikely to produce intoxication or any significant adverse behavioral effects. On the other hand, for people who are not tolerant to nicotine, it is probable that initial use of some products could produce intoxication.[41] The least likely delivery method to be capable of producing intoxication appears to be the transdermal systems, the nicotine vapor inhaler, and nicotine polacrilex, although for different reasons. The transdermal systems can deliver up to 22 mg of nicotine per day, but average only 0.9 mg/hour.[56,57] The nicotine vapor inhaler has such limited nicotine bioavailability that it would require approximately 100–200 puffs to obtain the 1–2 mg of nicotine typically obtained by taking 10 puffs from a cigarette.[35,58] Similarly, even the high dose of nicotine gum (labeled as 4 mg) requires 10–20 minutes of chewing to deliver 2–3 mg of nicotine.[32] In contrast, nicotine nasal spray could easily and rapidly be repeatedly administered to produce high levels of nicotine, although the nasal burning sensations produced by such behavior would presumably discourage most people from adopting this as a preferred means to produce intoxication.[9,58]

The variation in dosing capabilities in nicotine-delivering medications is a factor that has been considered by the Food and Drug Administration and its advisory committees in their deliberations concerning the approvability and level of marketing restrictions for nicotine.[23,24] If medications that provide even more rapid and less aversive means of delivering nicotine are developed, there is an increased risk that they would be used to produce intoxication and dependence in non-nicotine users.

Is nicotine a performance and learning enhancing drug?

There is increasing evidence that nicotine enhances learning and memory in animal models,[59,60] but the relevance of these findings to humans is not clear.[10,44] Results of studies conducted with nicotine-deprived smokers are difficult to interpret. Without pre-deprivation baseline data, which few studies report, it is difficult to conclude whether nicotine reverses deprivation-induced deficits or enhances performance beyond that observed in the nonabstinent state. In general, however, nicotine administration can reverse deprivation-induced behavioral deficits occurring in abstinent smokers, though such beneficial effects have not been observed consistently across a range of performance measures.[39] There is also preliminary evidence that nicotine can improve some aspects of memory in patients with Alzheimer's disease.[61,62]

The strongest conclusions concerning the effects of nicotine and smoking on human performance can be drawn from studies conducted with nondeprived smokers and nonsmokers. These studies have shown that nicotine enhanced finger tapping rate[14,63] and motor responding in tests of focused and divided attention.[64,65] On the basis of more limited evidence, nicotine produced faster motor responses on tests of visual scanning and memory[66,67] and on sustained attention.[68]

In an earlier commentary, Henningfield[44] addressed the question of whether nicotine was appropriately categorized as a performance enhancer and noted that "the purported benefits of nicotine self-administration have been the subject of scientific and medical debate during much of the twentieth century, with much of the focus on determining whether nicotine is a cognitive enhancer."[69,70] In that commentary, Henningfield[44] suggested reframing "the focus of scientific inquiry from attempting to determine which position is true to characterizing the effects of nicotine on a variety of measures to determine the conditions under which nicotine impairs performance and those under which it produces clinically meaningful cognitive benefits." It would take extraordinary, and heretofore undemonstrated, beneficial effects of nicotine delivered by tobacco on performance to justify exposure to the known risks of tobacco to people as a means of obtaining those benefits. In light of current evidence, it would also be difficult to justify nicotine medication use for its beneficial effects on performance except as a means of enabling formerly tobacco-dependent people to sustain their performance in the absence of tobacco. To this end, Henningfield[44] recommended that it remains important to "determine the conditions, if any, under which nicotine produces clinically meaningful cognitive benefits, as well as to define the range of conditions under which nicotine impairs cognition" and "to investigate the interaction between the cognitive effects of nicotine and the addiction potential of cigarettes."

Potential indirect effects of nicotine on performance

One characteristic of drug dependence is the degree to which preoccupation with self-administration of a substance can interfere with important activities.[25] There has been little systematic study of this phenomenon with respect to nicotine. To the extent to which it is important, and this will require systematic study, it could be hypothesized that the effect would be the worst with short-acting drug delivery systems that cannot be readily re-administered. An extreme case would be an oxygen-taking fighter pilot or brain surgeon dependent on tobacco who was required to undergo many hours of extremely demanding performance without the ability to readily re-administer the drug. In such cases, the early onset of withdrawal symptoms and the tendency to think more about the cigarette than the task at hand might lead to impaired performance. On the other hand, a delivery system such as a nicotine transdermal patch, which would deliver continuous nicotine, would not be as liable to these types of performance deficits.

Conclusions

The primary adverse behavioral effects of nicotine are related to its abuse liability and physical dependence potential (Chapter 12). The abuse liability can lead to maladaptive and harmful use, such as chronic tobacco self-administration. The physical dependence potential can contribute to this behavior because of the withdrawal symptoms that will likely occur after termination of nicotine intake. The abuse liability and dependence potential are most severe with cigarettes and much less severe with current nicotine-delivering medications (Chapter 12).

Although nicotine can directly disrupt performance and produce intoxication, these effects are relatively rare due to the development of tolerance and to the nature of the current dosing systems. Nonetheless, there is the potential for rapid delivering systems to produce intoxication, especially in nontolerant persons. Similarly, whereas the physical dependence potential is sufficient to enable nicotine-delivering medications to reduce nicotine withdrawal symptoms that accompany tobacco abstinence, withdrawal symptoms from the nicotine medications are generally lower, more tolerable, and more readily managed by gradual dose reduction. The primary beneficial effect of nicotine on performance and learning is to reverse or prevent the degradation that often accompanies tobacco withdrawal symptoms. Although nicotine can improve performance under certain conditions, the generality and clinical significance of these effects require further exploration to justify nicotine use on this basis.[39]

Acknowledgments

The authors appreciate Lakshmi Gopalan for her assistance in the preparation of this manuscript.

References

1. Miller NS (ed): *Principles of Addiction Medicine.* Chevy Chase, MD: American Society of Addiction Medicine, 1994.
2. Tashkin DP, Coulson AH, Clark VA, Simmons M, Bourque LB, Duann S, Spivey GH, Gong H: Respiratory symptoms and lung function in habitual heavy smokers of marijuana alone, smokers of marijuana and tobacco, smokers of tobacco alone, and nonsmokers. *American Review of Respiratory Diseases* 1987, 135:209–216.
3. Brookoff D, Cook CS, Williams C, Mann CS: Testing reckless drivers for cocaine and marijuana. *New England Journal of Medicine* 1994, 331:518–522.
4. Robbe HWJ: Influence of marijuana on driving. In Maastricht: University of Limburg Press, 1994.
5. O'Brien CP: Drug addiction and drug abuse. In Molinoff PB, Ruddon RW (eds): *Goodman and Gilman's The Pharmacological Basis of Therapeutics,* 9th ed. New York: McGraw-Hill, 1996, pp 557–575.
6. McGinnis JM, Foege WH: Actual causes of death in the United States. *Journal of the American Medical Association* 1993, 270:2207–2212.
7. Henningfield JE, Keenan RM: Nicotine delivery kinetics and abuse liability. *Journal of Consulting and Clinical Psychology* 1993, 61:743–750.
8. Heishman SJ, Kozlowski LT, Henningfield JE: Nicotine addiction: Implications for public health policy. *Journal of Social Issues* 1997, 53:13–33.
9. de Wit H, Zacny J: Abuse potential of nicotine replacement therapies. *Cent Nerv Syst Drugs* 1995, 4:456–468.
10. U.S. Department of Health and Human Services, Public Health Service: *The Health Consequences of Smoking: Nicotine Addiction* A report of the Surgeon General. Washington, DC: U.S. Government Printing Office, 1988.
11. Slade J: Nicotine delivery devices. In Orleans CT, Slade J (eds): *Nicotine Addiction: Principles and Management.* New York: Oxford University Press, 1993, pp 3–23.
12. Langley JN: On the reaction of cells and of nerve endings to certain poisons, chiefly as regards the reaction of striated muscle to nicotine and to currai. *Journal of Physiology* 1905, 33:374–413.
13. Swedberg MBD, Henningfield JE, Goldberg SR: Nicotine dependency: Animal studies. In Wonnacott S, Russell MAH, Stolerman IP (eds): *Nicotine Pharmacology: Molecular, Cellular and Behavioral Aspects.* Oxford: Oxford University Press, 1990, pp 38–75.
14. Perkins KA, Grobe JE, Fonte C, Goettler J, Caggiula AR, Reynolds WA, Stiller RL, Scierka A, Jacob RG: Chronic and acute tolerance to subjective, behavioral and cardiovascular effects of nicotine in humans. *Journal of Pharmacology and Experimental Therapeutics* 1994, 270:628–638.
15. Benowitz NL: Pharmacokinetic considerations in understanding nicotine dependence.

In Bock G, Marsh J (eds): *The Biology of Nicotine Dependence.* Wiley: Chichester, 1990, pp 186–209.

16. Pickworth WB, Bunker EB, Henningfield JE: Transdermal nicotine: Reduction of smoking with minimal abuse liability. *Psychopharmacology* 1994, 115:9–14.
17. Soria R, Stapleton JM, Gilson SF, Sampson-Cone A, Henningfield JE, London ED: Subjective and cardiovascular effects of intravenous nicotine in smokers and non-smokers. *Psychopharmacology* 1996, 128:221–226.
18. Sheiner LB: Clinical pharmacology and the choice between theory and empiricism. *Clinical Pharmacology and Therapeutics* 1989, 46:605–615.
19. Henningfield JE, Stapleton JM, Benowitz NL, London ED: Higher levels of nicotine in arterial than in venous blood after cigarette smoking. *Drug and Alcohol Dependence* 1993, 33:23–29.
20. Gourlay SG, Benowitz NL: Arteriovenous differences in plasma concentrations of nicotine and catecholamines and related cardiovascular effects after smoking, nicotine nasal spray, and intrevenous nicotine. *Clinical Pharmocology and Therapeutics* 1997, 62: 453–463.
21. Henningfield JE, Radzius A, Cone E: Estimation of available nicotine content of six smokeless tobacco products. *Tobacco Control* 1995, 4:57–61.
22. Djordjevic MV, Hoffman D, Glynn T, Connolly G: U.S. commercial brands of moist snuff, 1994. I. Assessment of nicotine, moisture and pH. *Tobacco Control* 1995, 4: 62–66.
23. Food and Drug Administration: 21 CFR Part 801, et al. Regulations Restricting Sale and Distribution of Cigarettes and Smokeless Tobacco Products to Protect Children and Adolescents. Proposed Rule. *Federal Register,* Friday, August 11, 1995, (60)155.
24. Food and Drug Administration: 21 CFR Part 801, et al. Regulations Restricting the Sale and Distribution of Cigarettes and Smokeless Tobacco Products to Protect Children and Adolescents. Final Rule. *Federal Register,* Wednesday, August 28, 1996, (61)168.
25. American Psychiatric Association: *Diagnostic and Statistical Manual of Mental Disorders,* 4th ed (DSM IV). Washington, DC: American Psychiatric Association, 1994.
26. Hughes JR, Higgins ST, Hatsukami D: Effects of abstinence from tobacco. In Kozlowski LT, Annis HM, Cappel HD, Glaser FB, Goodstadt MS, Israel Y, Kalant H, Sellers EM, Vingilis ER (eds): *Research Advances in Alcohol and Drug Problems.* New York: Plenum, 1990, pp 317–398.
27. Fiore MC, Shi FY, Heishman SJ, Henningfield JE: *The Effect of Smoking and Smoking Withdrawal on Flight Performance: A 1994 Update.* Atlanta: Centers for Disease Control and Prevention, 1994.
28. Jaffe JH: Drug addiction and drug abuse. In Gilman AG, Rall TW, Nies AS, Taylor P (eds): Goodman and Gilman's *The Pharmacological Basis of Therapeutics,* 8h ed. New York: Pergamon Press, 1990, pp 522–573.
29. Sachs DPL, Säwe U, Leischow SJ: Effectiveness of a 16-hour transdermal nicotine patch in a medical practice setting, without intensive group counseling. *Archives of Internal Medicine* 1993, 153:1881–1890.
30. Pickworth WB, Heishman SJ, Henningfield JE: Relationships between EEG and performance during nicotine withdrawal and administration. In Domino EF (ed): *Brain Imaging of Nicotine and Tobacco Smoking.* Ann Arbor: NPP Books, 1995, pp 275–287.
31. Hatsukami DK, Gust SW, Keenan RM: Physiologic and subjective changes from smokeless tobacco withdrawal. *Clinical Pharmacology and Therapeutics* 1987, 41: 103–107.

32. Benowitz NL, Porchet H, Sheiner L, Jacob P: Nicotine absorption and cardiovascular effects with smokeless tobacco use: Comparison with cigarettes and nicotine gum. *Clinical Pharmacology and Therapeutics* 1988, 44:23–28.

33. Fiore MC, Smith SS, Jorenby DE, Baker T: The effectiveness of the nicotine patch for smoking cessation, a meta-analysis. *Journal of the American Medical Association* 1994, 271:1940–1947.

34. Dubois JP, Sioufi A, Müller PH, Mauli D, Imhof PR: Pharmacokinetics and bioavailability of nicotine in healthy volunteers following single and repeated administration of different doses of transdermal nicotine systems. *Methods and Findings in Experimental and Clinical Pharmacology* 1989, 11:187–195.

35. Henningfield JE: Nicotine medications for smoking cessation. *New England Journal of Medicine* 1995, 333:1196–1203.

36. American Psychiatric Association: Practice Guideline for the Treatment of Patients with Nicotine Dependence. *American Journal of Psychiatry* 1996, 153(suppl):1–31.

37. Fiore MC, Bailey WC, Cohen SJ, et al.: *Smoking Cessation.* Clinical Practice Guideline No. 18. Rockville, MD: U.S. Department of Health and Human Services, Public Health Service, Agency for Health Care Policy and Research Publication No. 96-0692, April 1996.

38. Henningfield JE: Behavioral pharmacology of cigarette smoking. In Thompson T, Dews PB, Barrett JE (eds): *Advances in Behavioral Pharmacology,* vol IV. New York: Academic Press, 1984, pp 131–210.

39. Heishman SJ, Taylor RC, Henningfield JE: Nicotine and smoking: A review of effects on human performance. *Experimental Clinical Psychopharmacology* 1994, 2: 345–395.

40. Stolerman IP, Bunker P, Jarvik ME: Nicotine tolerance in rats: Role of dose and dose interval. *Pyschopharmacologia* (Berlin) 1974, 34:317–324.

41. Heishman SJ, Snyder FR, Henningfield JE: Performance, subjective and physiological effects of nicotine in nonsmokers. *Drug and Alcohol Dependence* 1993, 34:11–18.

42. Snyder FR, Henningfield JE: Effects of nicotine administration following 12 hours of tobacco deprivation: Assessment on computerized performance tasks. *Psychopharmacology* 1989, 97:17–22.

43. Carroll ME, Lac ST, Asencio M, Keenan RM: Nicotine dependence in rats. *Life Science* 1989, 45:1381–1388.

44. Henningfield JE: Do the benefits of nicotine help cigarettes beat the addiction rap? *Addiction* 1994, 89:135–146.

45. Perkins KA, Epstein LH, Stiller RL, Sexton JE, Debski TD, Jacob RG: Behavioral performance effects of nicotine in smokers and nonsmokers. *Pharmacology, Biochemistry, and Behavior* 1990, 37:11–15.

46. Pickworth WB, Fant RV, Butschky MF, Henningfield JE: Effects of transdermal nicotine delivery on measures of acute nicotine withdrawal. *Journal of Pharmacology and Experimental Therapeutics* 1996, 279:450–456.

47. Stolerman IP, Goldfarb T, Fink R, Jarvik ME: Influencing cigarette smoking with nicotine antagonists. *Psychopharmacologia* (Berlin) 1973, 28:247–259.

48. Clarke PBS, Kumar R: Nicotine does not improve discrimination of brain stimulation reward by rats. *Psychopharmacology* 1983, 79:271–277.

49. Jarvik ME: Commentary. *Psychopharmacology* 1995, 117:18–20.

50. Casey K: *If Only I Could Quit: Becoming a Nonsmoker.* Centercity: Hazelden Books, 1987.

51. Wilbert J: The ethnopharmacology of tobacco in native South America. Effects of

nicotine on biological systems. *Advances in Pharmacological Sciences.* Basel: Birk-häuser Verlag, 1991, pp 7–16.

52. *Physicians' Desk Reference,* 51st ed. Montvale: Medical Economics Company, 1997.
53. Tomar SL, Giovino GA, Eriksen MP: Smokeless tobacco brand preference and brand switching among U.S. adolescents and young adults. *Tobacco Control* 1995, 4:67–72.
54. Slade J: Are tobacco products drugs? Evidence from U.S. tobacco. *Tobacco Control* 1995, 4:1–2.
55. Henningfield JE, Kozlowski LT, Benowitz NL: A proposal to develop a meaningful labeling for cigarettes. *Journal of the American Medical Association* 1994, 272: 312–314.
56. Benowitz NL: Nicotine replacement therapy: What has been accomplished—Can we do better? *Drugs* 1993, 45:157–170.
57. Fagerström KO, Säwe U, Tonnesen: Therapeutic use of nicotine patches: Efficacy and safety. *Journal of Smoking Related Disease* 1992, 3:247–261.
58. Schuh JK, Schuh LM, Henningfield JE, Stitzer ML: Nicotine nasal spray and vapor inhaler: Abuse liability assessment. *Psychopharmacology* 1997, 130:352–361.
59. Arendash GW, Sanberg PR, Sengstock GJ: Nicotine enhances the learning and memory of aged rats. *Pharmacology, Biochemistry, and Behavior* 1995, 52:517–523.
60. Levin ED: Nicotine systems and cognitive function. *Psychopharmacology* 1992, 108: 417–431.
61. Jones GMM, Sahakian BJ, Levy R, Warburton DM, Gray JA: Effects of acute subcutaneous nicotine on attention, information processing and short-term memory in Alzheimer's disease. *Psychopharmacology* 1992, 108:485–494.
62. Newhouse PA, Sunderland T, Tariot PN, Blumhardt CL, Weingartner H, Mellow A, Murphy DL: Intravenous nicotine in Alzheimer's disease: A pilot study. *Psychopharmacology* 1988, 95:171–175.
63. West RJ, Jarvis MJ: Effects of nicotine on finger tapping rate in non-smokers. *Pharmacology, Biochemistry, and Behavior* 1986, 25:727–731.
64. Le Houezec J, Halliday R, Benowitz NL, Callaway E, Naylor H, Herzig K: A low dose of subcutaneous nicotine improves information processing in non-smokers. *Psychopharmacology* 1994, 114:628–634.
65. Sherwood N, Kerr JS, Hindmarch I: Psychomotor performance in smokers following single and repeated doses of nicotine gum. *Psychopharmacology* 1992, 108:432–436.
66. Kerr JS, Sherwood N, Hindmarch I: Separate and combined effects of the social drugs on psychomotor performance. *Psychopharmacology* 1991, 104:113–119.
67. West R, Hack S: Effect of cigarettes on memory search and subjective ratings. *Pharmacology, Biochemistry, and Behavior* 1991, 38:281–286.
68. Foulds J, Stapleton J, Swettenham J, Bell N, McSorley K, Russell MAH: Cognitive performance effects of subcutaneous nicotine in smokers and never-smokers. *Psychopharmacology* 1996, 127:31–38.
69. Bates RL: The effects of cigar and cigarette smoking on certain psychological and physiological functions: I. Dart throwing. *Journal of Comparative Psychology* 1922, 2:371–423.
70. West R: Beneficial effects of nicotine: Fact or fiction? *Addiction* 1993, 88:589–590.
71. Pickworth WB, Keenan RM, Henningfield JE: Nicotine: Effects and mechanisms. In Chang LW, Dyer RS (eds): *Handbook of Neurotoxicology.* New York: Marcel Dekker, 1995, pp 801–824.

Chapter **14**

Dependence on and Abuse of Nicotine Replacement Medications: An Update

JOHN R. HUGHES

The terms *dependence* and *abuse* can be used in reference to premarket testing ("dependence/abuse potential/liability") and also to clinical syndromes. Abuse and dependence syndromes have well-accepted definitions in the World Health Organization's *International Classification of Diseases,* 10th edition (ICD-10)[1] and the American Psychiatric Association's *Diagnostic and Statistical Manual,* 4th edition (DSM-IV).[2]

The essential features of dependence in both the ICD-10 and DSM-IV are tolerance, withdrawal symptoms, and compulsive drug taking.[1,2] DSM-IV also defines *physiological dependence* (also known as *physical dependence*) as the presence of tolerance or withdrawal symptoms and distinguishes *dependence* with and without *physiological dependence*.[2] The essential feature of *abuse* in DSM-IV[2] and *harmful use* in ICD-10[1] is recurrent and significant adverse consequences related to repeated use. Behavioral phenomena used to make diagnoses of dependence and abuse are listed in Table 14-1. Another common term is *misuse*. This is typically defined as use of a drug for reasons other than those intended by the manufacturer or prescriber.[3]

There is evidence that nicotine replacement medications can induce the specific phenomena described above (i.e., tolerance, withdrawal, compulsive use, abuse, and misuse). This chapter updates previous reviews of this issue.[4-6]

Table 14-1. DSM-IV and ICD-10 Criteria for Dependence and Abuse Syndromes

DSM-IV	ICD-10
Physiological Dependence	
Tolerance	Tolerance
Withdrawal	Withdrawal
Compulsive Use	
Use more than intended	Strong desire or compulsion to use
Inability to stop or control use	Difficulties controlling onset, termination or levels of use
Great deal of time to obtain, use, or recover from use	Increased time to obtain, use or recover from use
Give up activities to use	Neglect of alternate interests
Use despite knowing use is harmful	Use despite evidence of harm
Abuse/Harm Use	
Continued use despite social or interpersonal problems from use	Pattern of use that damages physical or mental health
Legal problems from use	
Use in hazardous situations	
Use results in failure to fulfill obligations	

Tolerance

Both acute tolerance (i.e., occurring within a single or a few doses of the drug) and chronic tolerance (i.e., occurring after several doses) to the effects of nicotine readily occur during regular cigarette smoking.[7] Acute tolerance to nicotine itself, when given intravenously, has been documented.[8] With nicotine nasal spray, acute tolerance to subjective and cardiovascular effects has been repeatedly demonstrated.[9] Whether chronic use of nasal spray induces chronic tolerance has not been studied. Neither acute nor chronic tolerance has been studied in experiments with nicotine gum, patch, or inhaler.

Clinical observations suggest that during the first 1–2 weeks of use most patients develop tolerance to the aversive effects of nicotine gum, patch, nasal spray, and inhaler, including central nervous system aversive effects. As for longer term tolerance, two studies of nicotine nasal spray showed that the amount of use per day increased over time among long-term users, suggesting that tolerance was occurring.[10,11] However, two other studies did not find this pattern.[12,13] The two positive studies did not provide sufficient data to distinguish whether the dose escalation was due to a diminution of positive central nervous system effects or to a diminution of aversive peripheral effects. Escalation of dosing with transdermal nicotine or nicotine inhaler has not been reported. Use of nicotine gum decreases, rather than increases, over time.[14,15]

Withdrawal

Abrupt cessation of cigarettes and smokeless tobacco often produces a withdrawal syndrome.[16,17] In terms of nicotine replacement, abrupt cessation of nicotine gum can produce withdrawal symptoms similar to, but less intense than, that of smoking cessation.[5,6,18,19,20] The milder withdrawal may be due to the different rates of absorption of nicotine via cigarettes versus gum. Two studies showed a slight trend for more withdrawal to occur with 4 mg than with 2 mg gum.[18,20] The single empirical study found little difference in withdrawal from nicotine gum after chewing gum for 1 versus 3 months.[19] An across-study comparison suggests withdrawal is more intense in those who have found it necessary to use nicotine gum long term.[18] Finally, two studies suggested withdrawal from nicotine gum is more intense in women than in men.[19,18] Unfortunately, no studies have examined population-based estimates of the incidence or prevalence of nicotine gum withdrawal, whether withdrawal from nicotine gum prompts relapse to smoking or long-term use of nicotine gum, or whether withdrawal from gum is severe enough to be clinically significant.

Although three of the four transdermal nicotine systems recommend gradual reduction, whether abrupt cessation of transdermal nicotine can induce withdrawal is unclear. Two studies presented graphs suggesting that abrupt cessation might slightly increase some symptoms; however, no statistical analyses were presented.[21,22] A third study presented graphical data suggesting no withdrawal,[23] but some withdrawal was noted clinically (R.D. Hurt, personal communication, 1996). Finally, a meta-analysis found no difference in quit rates between abrupt and gradual reduction of transdermal nicotine,[24] suggesting that if any withdrawal occurred after abrupt cessation it did not increase relapse. Whether abrupt cessation of nicotine nasal spray or inhaler would induce withdrawal has not been studied.

Compulsive use

No studies have addressed the DSM-IV or ICD-10 criteria concerning compulsive use (see Table 14-1) in persons using nicotine replacement medications. Several studies have examined long-term use of nicotine gum, which, as described below, may not be equivalent to compulsive use.

A meta-analysis of 24 studies[6] reported that, at 12 months, 22% of those who had stopped smoking and received nicotine gum were continuing to use the gum compared with 7% of those who received placebo gum (Fig. 14-1). Comparable figures, based on all smokers prescribed the gum (intent-to-treat analysis) were 9% versus 4%. In addition, across the nine prospective or retrospective studies that had 2-year follow-up periods, a median of 3% of all those prescribed the gum were using nicotine gum (Housley and Sawell, unpublished data).[25-32] The fre-

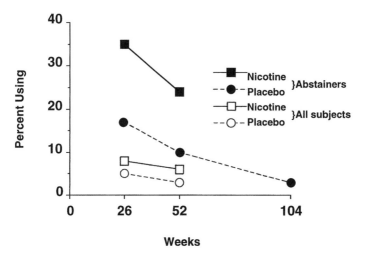

Figure 14-1. Incidence of use of nicotine gum in prospective studies. (Data from Hughes et al.[15])

quency of use (pieces per day) decreased over time in all seven studies that examined this.[6] At the 6–12-month follow up, the mean daily intake of gum was 15 mg (range, 10–22 mg/day).[6]

Instances of long-term use of nicotine patches have not been reported. Studies of nicotine nasal spray reported 32% and 43% of those abstinent, and 13% and 18% of all subjects were using nasal spray 6 months after cessation.[11–13] Two studies reported an increase in number of sprays per day at 1-, 3-, or 6-month follow ups,[10,11] but two other studies did not find this.[12,13] Whether nicotine inhaler is used long term has not been studied.

The incidence and prevalence figures for long-term use cited in the above text are probably overestimates as many studies did not charge for medications or discourage long-term use. In addition, the studies did not require subjects to use the medication on a daily basis to be counted as long-term users.[5]

Both the meta-analysis[6] and an experimental study[17] indicate that long-term use is not greater with 4 mg than with 2 mg gum. Both correlational[33] and experimental[34] studies indicate that increased cost substantially decreases long-term use. One might expect that smokers with high levels of nicotine dependence or a past history of alcohol or illicit drug dependence would have a higher incidence of long-term use, but this has not been found.[5] Also, ad libitum or as needed use of a drug might be expected to increase long-term use due to enrollment of conditioning factors; however, whether long-term use differs between ad libitum and scheduled use has not been studied. Expectancies about gum influence gum use in the first few weeks after cessation,[5] but whether these would influence long-term use has not been assessed. The fact that 4%–6% of those assigned placebo gum continued to use it for 6–12 months (see Fig. 14-1) suggests that some long-term use is due to expectancy effects. While no empirical data are available, clinical observations are that using nicotine patches long term has not been a problem. Whether persons with nicotine nasal spray or inhaler use these products long term has not been reported.

Demonstration of long-term use of a drug is not equivalent to demonstration of drug dependence (e.g., consider long-term daily use of caffeine).[35] As described above, a drug dependence syndrome is exemplified by, among other things, an inability to stop using a drug despite serious attempts to stop.[1,2] While studies have not directly posed these questions to patients using nicotine replacement, two sets of data indirectly test for a dependence syndrome.

One indication of dependence might be continued use of a medication after a physician has recommended stopping it. The above-referenced meta-analysis[5] located 11 studies in which such a stop date was given to subjects (3–4 months after cessation). In these studies, 33% of the subjects using nicotine gum continued to use the gum for 6 months (i.e., 2–3 months beyond the recommended stop date). Similar figures for nicotine patch, nasal spray, or inhaler are not available.

Another indication of dependence is difficulty in stopping the drug. In one study, 38% of those on nicotine gum and 25% of those on placebo stated that it was moderately to very difficult to stop using the gum.[6] On the other hand, in the three trials of treatments for cessation of long-term use of nicotine gum, simple instructions or placebo substitution have been adequate for the majority of patients.[36–38] In addition, simply having subjects pay for their gum substantially decreased long-term use in one trial.[34]

If long-term use is not dependence, how can one account for it? One possibility is that long-term users are simply trying to extend the duration of treatment. The recommended 3-month duration of therapy was not based on any experimental data, and many patients and clinicians believe therapy longer than 3 months is more helpful. Another possibility is that most of those who have stopped with the aid of nicotine replacement have a history of several failures at smoking cessation; thus, many of those abstinent from smoking and using nicotine gum long term may extend their treatment because they fear that stopping use of the gum will jeopardize their abstinence from cigarettes.

Abuse

A clinical syndrome of abuse of nicotine replacement requires that harm occurs from its use. Reports of significant medical or psychosocial harm from use of nicotine replacement are extremely rare.[39] This is because, unlike cigarette smoking, use of nicotine replacement medications produces no carbon monoxide or carcinogens. In addition, nicotine levels from medications are much less than those from smoking and occur as a result of a few episodes of slow onset of nicotine rather than from many episodes of rapid onset of nicotine.

Misuse

Although nicotine has a reputation of aiding in weight control or concentration, the use of nicotine replacement products by never-smokers has been quite rare, even when products are available over the counter.[28] The other, more common, misuse scenario is when smokers use nicotine replacement not to stop but rather to cut down on smoking or comply with smoking restrictions. The prevalence of persons concurrently smoking and using nicotine gum varied from 25% to 38% in three studies.[6,13,27] The comparable range for six studies of nicotine patch was 10%–54%.[40–45] Figures for nicotine nasal spray and inhaler are not available.

In experimental studies of concurrent smoking and gum or patch use in smokers not trying to quit smoking, smoking behavior decreased in all five studies and carbon monoxide levels decreased in four of five studies, suggesting decreased exposure to carcinogens and toxins (see Fig. 14-2).[46–52] However, nicotine levels increased in four of six studies.[46,47,51,52] Although there are fewer studies, similar results occurred with concomitant smoking and use of nicotine patch in smokers not trying to stop smoking.[53–55]

In evaluating the nicotine levels in these studies, one must remember these studies examined venous levels. It is unlikely that concomitant users would have higher arterial nicotine levels than those shown with smoking.[56] In addition, even if the blood nicotine levels are similar, the harm from many repeated boluses of nicotine, as in smoking, may be greater than harm from a few, slow-onset doses of nicotine. Only one study has examined medical harm from long-term concurrent smoking and use of nicotine replacement. This large, prospective trial did not find any evidence of increased cardiovascular risk from concurrent smoking and nicotine gum use (see Chapter 17).

Conclusions

Whether long-term use of nicotine replacement products produces chronic tolerance has not been determined. Abrupt cessation of nicotine gum can cause withdrawal, but substantially less withdrawal than is seen with cessation of cigarette smoking. Abrupt cessation of transdermal nicotine appears to produce little, if any, withdrawal. Withdrawal from nasal spray and inhaler has not been tested.

Long-term use of nicotine gum and nicotine nasal spray, but not transdermal nicotine, occurs in a small proportion of abstinent smokers. Whether long-term use of inhaler occurs has not been tested. Over time, the daily use of nicotine gum

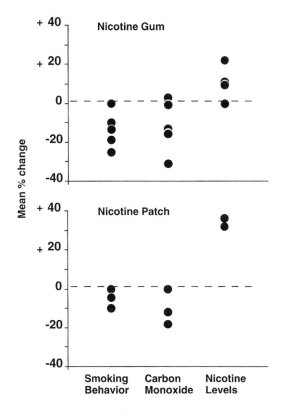

Figure 14-2. Effect of nicotine gum (**top**) and nicotine patch (**bottom**) on smoking in smokers not trying to quit smoking.

decreases. Whether the daily use of nasal spray increases or decreases over time is unclear. However, long-term use is not necessarily synonymous with dependence. Although some people may have a clinically significant dependence on gum or nasal spray, most seem to be extending the duration of their treatment—not developing dependence.

Evidence of nicotine replacement product abuse is essentially nonexistent. The major form of misuse is concurrent use of nicotine replacement and tobacco in smokers. Such use usually results in less smoking and less carbon monoxide, which suggests less exposure to carcinogens and other toxins. However, concurrent use often results in higher nicotine levels. Whether these higher nicotine levels are harmful has not been well studied.

Future research is needed to determine whether tolerance occurs to the beneficial effects of nicotine replacement and whether there is withdrawal from nasal spray and inhaler. In addition, more studies need to examine the clinical indices of dependence (e.g., difficulty stopping) on nicotine replacement. Finally, trials are needed to see whether toxin exposure and health harm occur from concurrent use of tobacco and nicotine replacement products.

References

1. World Health Organization: *International Classification of Diseases and Related Health Problems,* 10th ed. Geneva: World Health Organization. 1995.
2. American Psychiatric Association: *Diagnostic and Statistical Manual of Mental Disorders,* 4th ed. Washington, DC: American Psychiatric Association, 1994.
3. World Health Organization: Nomenclature and classification of drug and alcohol-related problems: A WHO memorandum. *Bulletin of the World Health Organization* 1981, 59:225–242.
4. de Wit H, Zacny JP: Abuse potential of nicotine replacement therapies. *Cent Nerv Syst Drugs* 1995, 4:456–468.
5. Hughes JR: Dependence potential and abuse liability of nicotine replacement therapies. *Biomedicine Pharmacotherapy* 1989, 43:11–17.
6. Hughes JR: Long-term use of nicotine-replacement therapy. In Henningfield JE, Stitzer ML (eds): *New Developments in Nicotine-Delivery Systems.* New York: Carlton Publishers, 1991, pp 64–71.
7. U.S. Department of Health and Human Services: *The Health Consequences of Smoking: Nicotine Addiction.* A Report of the U.S. Surgeon General. Washington, DC: U.S. Government Printing Office, 1988.
8. Porchet HC, Benowitz NL, Sheiner LB: Pharmacodynamic model of tolerance: Application to nicotine. *Journal of Pharmacology and Experimental Therapeutics* 1988, 244:213–236.
9. Perkins KA, Grobe JE, Mitchell SL, Goettler J, Caggiula A, Stiller RL, Scierka A: Acute tolerence to nicotine in smokers: Lack of dissipation within 2 hours. *Psychopharmacology* 1995, 118:164–170.
10. Blondal T, Franzon M, Westin A, Olafsdottir I, Gudmundsdottir S, Gunnarsdottir R: Controlled trial of nicotine nasal spray with long term follow-up. American Lung Association/American Thoracic Society International Conference, San Francisco, California, May 17, 1993.
11. Sutherland G, Stapleton JA, Russell MAH, Jarvis MJ, Hajek P, Belcher M, Feyerabend C: Randomized controlled trial of nasal nicotine spray in smoking cessation. *Lancet* 1992, 340:324–329.
12. Hjalmarson A, Franzon M, Westin A, Wiklund O: Effect of nicotine nasal spray on smoking cessation. *Archives of Internal Medicine* 1994, 154:2567–2572.
13. Schneider NG, Olmstead R, Mody FV, Doan K, Franzon M, Jarvik ME, Steinberg C: Efficacy of a nicotine nasal spray in smoking cessation: A placebo-controlled, double-blind trial. *Addiction* 1995, 90:1671–1682.
14. Hughes JR: Environmental determinants of the reinforcing effects of nicotine. *Journal of Substance Abuse* 1:319–329.
15. Hughes JR, Gust SW, Keenan RM, Skoog K, Fenwick JW, Higgins ST: Long-term use of nicotine versus placebo gum. *Archives of Internal Medicine* 1991, 151:1993–1998.
16. Hughes JR, Hatsukami DK: The nicotine withdrawal syndrome: A brief review and update. *International Journal of Smoking Cessation* 1992, 1:21–26.
17. Hughes JR, Higgins ST, Hatsukami DK: Effects of abstinence from tobacco: A critical review. *Research Advances in Alcohol and Drug Problems* 1990, 10:317–398.

18. Hatsukami DK, Skoog K, Allen S, Bliss R: Gender and the effects of different doses of nictone gum on tobacco withdrawal symptoms. *Experimental and Clinical Psychopharmacology* 1995, 3:163–173.

19. Hatsukami DK, Huber M, Callies A, Skoog K: Physical dependence on nicotine gum: Effect of duration of use. *Psychopharmacology* 1993, 111:449–456.

20. Hatsukami DK, Skoog K, Huber M, Hughes JR: Signs and symptoms from nicotine gum abstinence. *Psychopharmacology* 1991, 104:496–504.

21. Fiore MC, Kenford SL, Jorenby DE, Wetter DW, Smith SS, Baker TB: Two studies of the clinical effectiveness of the nicotine patch with different counseling treatments. *Chest* 1994, 105:524–533.

22. Levin ED, Westman EC, Stein RM, Carnahan E, Sanchez M, Herman S, Behm FM, Rose JE: Nicotine skin patch treatment increases abstinence, decreases withdrawal symptoms and attenuates rewarding effects of smoking. *Journal of Clinical Psychopharmacology* 1994, 14:41–49.

23. Hurt RD, Dale LC, Fredrickson PA, Caldwell CC, Lee GA, Offord KP, Lauger GG, Marusic Z, Neese LW, Lundberg TG: Nicotine patch therapy for smoking cessation combined with physician advice and nurse follow-up. *Journal of the American Medical Association* 1994, 271:595–600.

24. Fiore MC, Smith SS, Jorenby DE, Baker TB: The effectiveness of the nicotine patch for smoking cessation: A meta-analysis. *Journal of the American Medical Association* 1994, 271:1940–1946.

25. Leo AB: *A Survey of Over-the-Counter Use of Nicotine Gum.* Helsingborg, Sweden: A.B. Leo, 1987.

26. Hjalmarson AI: Effect of nicotine chewing gum in smoking cessation. *Journal of the American Medical Association* 1984, 252:2835–2838.

27. Johnson RE, Stevens VJ, Hollis JF, Woodson GT: Nicotine chewing gum use in the outpatient care setting. *Journal of Family Practice* 1992, 34:61–65.

28. Ramstrom LM: Use of nicotine replacement therapy with and without prescription. In *Future Directions in Nicotine Replacement Therapy.* Chester, England: Adis, 1994, pp 28–34

29. Raw M, Jarvis MJ, Feyerabend C, Russell MAH: Comparison of nicotine chewing gum and psychological treatments for nicotine dependence. *British Medical Journal* 1980, 281:481–482.

30. Tonnesen P, Fryd V, Hansen M, Helsted J, Gunnersen A, Forchammer H, Stockner M: Effect of nicotine chewing gum in combination with group counseling in the cessation of smoking. *New England Journal of Medicine* 1988, 318:15–27.

31. Westling H: Experience with nicotine-containing chewing gum in smoking cessation. *Lakartidningen* 1976, 73:2549–2552.

32. Wilhelmsen L, Hjalmarson AI: Smoking cessation experience in Sweden. *Canadian Family Physician* 1980, 26:737–743.

33. Cox JL, McKenna JP: Nicotine gum: Does providing it free in a smoking cessation program alter success rates? *Journal of Family Practice* 1990, 31:278–280.

34. Hughes JR, Wadland WC, Fenwick JW, Lewis J, Bickel WK: Effect of cost on the self-administration and efficacy of nicotine gum: A preliminary study. *Preventive Medicine* 1991, 20:486–496.

35. Hughes JR, Oliveto AH, Helzer JE, Higgins ST, Bickel WK: Should caffeine abuse, dependence or withdrawal be added to DSM-IV or ICD-10? *American Journal of Psychiatry* 1992, 149:33–40.

36. Bittoun R: Coming off long-term nicotine gum. *Lancet* 1989, 2:1164.

37. Hurt RD, Offord KP, Lauger GG, Marusic Z, Fagerstrom K, Enright PL, Scanlon PD: Cessation of long-term nicotine gum use: A prospective, randomized trial. *Addiction* 1995, 90:407–413.
38. Waranch HR, Henningfield JE, Edmunds M: Elimination of nicotine gum use. *Lancet* 1988, 1:49–50.
39. Hughes JR: Risk/benefit of nicotine replacement in smoking cessation. *Drug Safety* 1993, 8:49–56.
40. Cummings KM, Biernbaum RM, Zevon MA, Deloughry T, Jaen C: Use and effectiveness of transdermal nicotine in primary care settings. *Archives of Family Medicine* 1994, 3:682–689.
41. Haxby D, Sinclair A, Eiff MP, McQueen MH, Toffler WL: Characteristics and perceptions of nicotine patch users. *Journal of Family Practice* 1994, 38:459–464.
42. Hines D, Humm R: Patient compliance with nicotine patch use in a community setting. Society of Behavioral Medicine Meeting, Boston, 1994.
43. Orleans CT, Resch N, Noll E, Keintz MK, Rimer BK, Brown TV, Snedden TM: Use of transdermal nicotine in a state-level prescription plan for the elderly. *Journal of the American Medical Association* 1994, 271:601–607.
44. Pierce JP, Gilpin E, Farkas AJ: Nicotine patch use in the general population: Results from the 1993 California Tobacco Survey. *Journal of the National Cancer Institute* 1995, 87:87–93.
45. Willey C, Laforge R, Prochaska J, Levesque D: Transdermal nicotine usage in a randomly selected population based sample of smokers. Society of Behavioral Medicine Meeting, San Diego, 1995.
46. Ebert RV, McNabb ME, Snow SL: Effect of nicotine chewing gum on plasma nicotine levels of cigarette smokers. *Clinical Pharmacology and Therapeutics* 1994, 35: 495–498.
47. Herning RI, Jones RT, Fischman P: The titration hypothesis revisted: Nicotine gum reduces smoking intensity. In Grabowski J, Hall SM (eds): *Pharmacological Adjuncts in Smoking Cessation.* National Institute on Drug Abuse Research Monograph 53. Washington, DC: U.S. Government Printing Office, 1985, pp 27–41.
48. Kozlowski LT, Jarvik ME, Gritz ER: Nicotine regulations and cigarette smoking. *Clinical Pharmacology and Therapeutics* 1974, 17:93–97.
49. Nemeth-Coslett R, Henningfield JE, O'Keefe MK, Griffiths RR: Effects of mecamylamine on human cigarette smoking and subjective ratings. *Psychopharmacology* 1986, 88:420–425.
50. Nemeth-Coslett R, Henningfield JE: Effects of nicotine chewing gum on cigarette smoking and subjective and physiologic effects. *Clinical Pharmacology and Therapeutics* 1986, 39:625–630.
51. Russell MAH, Sutton SR, Feyerabend C, Cole PV: Effect of nicotine chewing gum on smoking behavior and as an aid to cigarette withdrawal. *British Medical Journal* 1976, 2:391–393.
52. Turner JAMcM, Taylor DM, Sillett RW, McNicol MW: The effects of supplementary nicotine in regular cigarette smokers. *Postgraduate Medical Journal* 1977, 53: 683–686.
53. Foulds J, Stapleton J, Feyerabend C, Vesey C, Jarvis M, Russell MAH: Effect of transdermal nicotine patches on cigarette smoking: A double-blind crossover study. *Psychopharmacology* 1992, 106:421–427.
54. Hartman N, Leong GB, Glynn SM, Wilkins JN, Jarvik ME: Transdermal nicotine and

smoking behavior in psychiatric patients. *American Journal of Psychiatry* 1991, 148: 374–375.

55. Pickworth WB, Bunker EB, Henningfield JE: Transdermal nicotine: Reduction of smoking with minimal abuse liability. *Psychopharmacology* 1994, 115:9–14.

56. Henningfield JE, Stapleton JM, Benowitz NL, Grayson RF, London ED: Higher levels of nicotine in arterial than in venous blood after cigarette smoking. *Drug and Alcohol Dependency* 1993, 33:23–29.

Other Topics

Cigarette smoking has been linked to gastrointestinal disease. Smokers have an increased risk of peptic ulcer disease and esophageal reflux, and smokers with peptic ulcer disease have a poor response to many acid-suppressing medications. On the other hand, smoking is protective against ulcerative colitis, and ulcerative colitis is more likely to appear for the first time when a smoker stops smoking. The first chapter of Part V explores how nicotine contributes to peptic ulcer disease and how nicotine may work to ameliorate ulcerative colitis. Also reviewed are data on the clinical use of nicotine as a medication to treat ulcerative colitis—the first clinical application of nicotine as a medication for other than smoking cessation.

A great deal of adverse drug reaction data have been collected from the United States Food and Drug Administration as part of ongoing, postmarketing surveillance. In Part V, the Food and Drug Administration adverse drug reaction data are reviewed.

Finally, the longest studied duration of use of nicotine medication in people is the use of nicotine gum in the Lung Health Study. In this study, some individuals used nicotine gum for up to 5 years. The safety data from this trial, including acute cardiovascular events and gastrointestinal disease, are the best data available on the long-term safety of nicotine.

Chapter 15

Nicotine and the Gastrointestinal Tract

JOHN RHODES, JOHN GREEN, and GARETH THOMAS

There is little information about the direct effects of nicotine on the gastrointestinal tract in humans. Most observations derive from studies of smoking. The effect of smoking on body weight is perhaps the best recognized observation, and it accounts for up to a 10% difference between smokers and nonsmokers.

Approximately 30 years ago, a former British medical officer recounted his experiences with troops who were prisoners of war during the Nazi occupation of Greece. The prisoners had very inadequate food rations and suffered severe hunger pains, which they tried to relieve in various ways. The only thing that consistently relieved the pain was smoking a cigarette. In the late 1930s, Schnedorf and Ivy[1] identified the basis for this observation in volunteers: Smoking inhibits the gastric contractions associated with hunger. Although the relevance of this to the weight of smokers is unknown, there are short-term changes in calorie intake with cessation and resumption of smoking, yet most studies show no difference in long-term calorie intake. Reduction in body weight with tobacco use may result from both decreased energy intake and increased energy expenditure.[2] Nicotine in rodents has been shown to reduce their food intake, increasing energy expenditure and decreasing weight. Conversely, nicotine withdrawal causes hyperphagia and weight gain.[3]

Smoking and peptic ulcer disease

Most of the interest in the gastrointestinal effects of smoking and nicotine has been related to peptic ulcer disease, as summarized in the U.S. Surgeon General's

1979 report. Patients with peptic ulcers, both duodenal and gastric, smoke more. The increased prevalence of peptic ulcer among smokers is related to the number of cigarettes smoked. In addition, smoking delays healing of duodenal and gastric ulcers and is associated with increased mortality in those with ulcer disease.

The mechanisms involved cause disruption of the normal balance between the erosive actions of acid and pepsin and the mucosal resistance. The roles of bile and bile acids in this equation are of interest because the detergent effect of bile damages the mucosal barrier. Reflux of bile into the stomach is a particular feature of gastric ulcer. In the late 1960s and early 1970s, it was shown that patients with esophagitis due to gastroesophageal reflux not only had an incompetent pylorus but also an incompetent gastroesophageal junction. Esophagitis is often caused by the combined damaging effect of both bile and acid. Reflux of bile at both sites is provoked by smoking.[4]

Transdermal nicotine's effect on gastroesophageal reflux

Recent observations of the effect of transdermal nicotine on gastroesophageal reflux have been made in volunteers, some of whom were smokers.[5] Volunteers wore placebo patches for 24 hours, followed by nicotine patches for the subsequent 24 hours; throughout this 48-hour time period, esophageal pH was monitored continuously. Gastroesophageal reflux causes a fall in the esophageal pH, but once acid has cleared from the esophagus the pH returns to neutral. Results showed that major differences occurred when subjects were supine: The number of episodes of acid reflux was greater, and the length of time the pH was acidic increased with nicotine. The practical implication would appear to be that nicotine patches should be removed at night to avoid unnecessary gastroesophageal reflux with damage to the lower esophagus.

The effect of smoking on duodenal ulcer

With the advent of H2 receptor antagonists in the 1970s, many clinical trials were conducted with duodenal ulcers that included data on the effect of smoking on healing and clinical relapse. Healing is delayed in smokers and is related to the number of cigarettes smoked.[6] Relapse from duodenal ulcer is also related to the number of cigarettes smoked, and there are important associations between relapse, smoking status, and treatment. Healing rates of duodenal ulcers, over a 4-week time period with cimetidine treatment, were highest in nonsmokers and lowest in those who smoked more than 30 cigarettes daily.[6] The cumulative relapse rate over a 12-month period was lowest in nonsmokers and highest in those smoking more than 30 cigarettes a day.[7] The recurrence of duodenal ulcer in smokers and nonsmokers given cimetidine or placebo showed the lowest recurrence in nonsmokers given cimetidine. The highest relapse rate occurred in smokers without the H2 antagonist. The nonsmokers given placebo fared almost as well as the smokers taking cimetidine—smoking almost totally undercut the therapeutic effect of cimetidine.

Nicotine and the mucous bicarbonate barrier

Mechanisms underlying the gastrointestinal effects of nicotine are probably related to the mucous bicarbonate barrier in the stomach. Details of this interaction have been explored in the last 15 years, but the issue was identified in Oxford, England, in the late 1950s by Heatley.[8] On the surface of gastric mucosal epithelium is a layer of adherent visible mucus into which bicarbonate is secreted. The layer of mucus acts as a barrier between epithelium and acid in the gastric lumen, with a gradient of pH through the mucous layer. Smoking—and possibly nicotine—decreases bicarbonate secretion,[9] which is related to endogenous prostaglandins in the mucosa; it may also increase acid secretion and thus disrupt the barrier. Smoking reduces the production of endogenous prostaglandins in gastric mucosa with an effect on both bicarbonate and mucous secretion and a possible increase in acid.[10] There is also evidence that smoking increases infection with *Helicobacter pylori,* an organism associated with peptic ulcer.

Other possible mechanisms have been suggested and include changes in the circulation, but there is a possibility that only one mechanism is principally involved. Work with nicotine itself in relation to peptic ulcer has been limited to animal models in which gastric ulceration induced by various chemicals is usually augmented by the concurrent administration of nicotine. A series of experiments were carried out in rabbits and ferrets given subcutaneous infusions of nicotine over a 2-week period. Measurements of the gastric mucus thickness and endogenous eicosanoids showed no significant change with nicotine.

Nicotine, esophageal reflux, and peptic ulcer disease

With respect to the effect of nicotine on esophageal reflux and peptic ulcer disease, it is noteworthy that several trials have been carried out in patients with ulcerative colitis, all of whom were nonsmokers. Half of the patients in each trial were given transdermal nicotine. Side effects were noted, and, although nausea and light-headedness were common, none of these patients spontaneously complained of epigastric discomfort or heartburn. Future trials need to address the relationship between transdermal nicotine and peptic ulcer in humans and answer specific questions about heartburn and epigastric discomfort.

Nicotine and ulcerative colitis

In 1982, an association between smoking and colitis was discovered.[11] Patients with Crohn's disease are often malnourished, and, in a study of nutritional status, we recorded anthropometric measurements using patients with ulcerative colitis as a control group. Because of the effect of smoking on body weight, the values from smokers and nonsmokers were examined. Surprisingly, results showed that almost all of those with ulcerative colitis were nonsmokers. At the time, 44% of the adult controls were smokers compared with only 8% of patients with colitis.[11]

Several groups in later studies assessed patients who were exsmokers with colitis. The time relationships between cessation of smoking and onset of colitis have been noted. One study showed that a total of 75% of these patients stopped smoking before the onset of their colitis; only a minority of patients developed colitis while still smoking. The incidence of colitis was especially high in both men and women in the early years after stopping smoking.[12]

An obvious question is whether smoking improves colitis or prevents relapse and, if so, through what mechanism. Reliable data on the effect of smoking on ulcerative colitis are difficult to obtain because controlled studies that involve stopping and starting smoking would be difficult to conduct and would breach ethical considerations. However, half of a group of 30 patients who were intermittent smokers noticed an improvement in symptoms over 6 weeks while smoking 20 cigarettes daily.[13]

Transdermal nicotine therapy for colitis

From a therapeutic point of view, the possibility that nicotine may be the active component was of interest because transdermal nicotine would overcome the practical difficulties of testing the effect of smoking. After various pilot studies, the effect of nicotine in three controlled trials was examined: two in acute colitis[14,15] and one as maintenance therapy.[16] A summary of findings showed that nicotine significantly benefited acute colitis when used in addition to conventional treatment with 5-amino salicylic acid or steroids. In a second study, it was used alone and compared with moderate doses of prednisolone; although it was of benefit, it was less effective than 15 mg of prednisolone.

As maintenance therapy for smoking cessation, nicotine or placebo patches were given to randomized patients who were then followed for 6 months. Most patients were given 15 mg of nicotine daily, but there was no significant difference between the groups followed, suggesting that, in this dose, nicotine was not of value as maintenance treatment.

The association of smoking and colitis

The mechanisms underlying the association of smoking and colitis remain an enigma, but various possibilities have been explored. Smoking causes a transient reduction in blood flow to the colonic mucosa and has an effect on oxygen-free radicals. Well-documented changes in cellular immunity associated with smoking have been examined in some detail, with some changes also in humoral immunity. However, there is some difficulty in identifying the immunological effect as the underlying mechanism when two closely related diseases, ulcerative colitis and Crohn's disease, show opposite effects with smoking. Changes occur in the mucosal eicosanoids and possibly in the colonic mucus, which may be part of the mechanism. However, after much effort, no causal mechanism has been identified.

Smoking and Crohn's disease

Crohn's disease is closely related to ulcerative colitis. However, in several respects the relationship to smoking is one of striking "opposites." Ulcerative colitis is a disease of nonsmokers, while Crohn's disease is principally a disease of smokers.[17] In Crohn's disease, there is evidence of an increased incidence related to passive exposure to smoke in childhood. In addition, patients who smoke heavily tend to have small bowel disease. There is also evidence that symptoms are made worse by smoking and that the number of surgical relapses is increased in smokers. In this respect, there are several long-term studies showing that the number of patients requiring further surgery is greater among smokers than nonsmokers.[18]

Nicotine and cardiovascular risk

Trials in ulcerative colitis have presented a unique opportunity to examine the effects of nicotine in nonsmokers. In the maintenance trial, consideration was given to whether nicotine was associated with increased cardiovascular risk. As a result, a series of measurements were taken in 20 patients given nicotine and 25 given placebo. This trial was randomized and double blind.[19] There is no "gold standard" to predict risk, but the measurements used are known to change in smokers. None, with the exception of fibrinogen, changed significantly. Fibrinogen has been used as an independent marker to predict cardiovascular events[20] and, surprisingly, showed a significant fall with nicotine. Fibrinogen increases in response to inflammation and its fall, may reflect a diminished inflammation secondary to nicotine treatment in patients with colitis. Again, this needs to be measured in future studies, particularly with nonsmokers so that changes are not confounded by smoking.

Conclusions

There are few direct observations on the effects of nicotine itself on the gastrointestinal tract. Transdermal nicotine provokes gastroesophageal reflux with heartburn. It also promotes healing in active ulcerative colitis, which is usually a disease of nonsmokers. Other associations with the gastrointestinal tract are indirect and depend on smoking observations.

References

1. Schnedorf JG, Ivy AC: The effect of tobacco smoking on the alimentary tract: An experimental study of man and animals. *Journal of the American Medical Association* 1939, 112:898–903.
2. Perkins KA: Metabolic effects of cigarette smoking. *Journal of Applied Physiology* 1992, 72:401–409.
3. Winders SE, Grunberg NE: Effects of nicotine on body weight, food consumption and body composition in male rats. *Life Sciences* 1990, 46:1523–1530.
4. Rees WDW, Rhodes J: Bile reflux in gastro oesophageal disease. *Clinics in Gastroenterology* 1977, 6:179–200.
5. Rahal PS, Wright RA: Transdermal nicotine and gastro-oesophageal reflux. *American Journal of Gastroenterology* 1995, 90:919–921.
6. Korman MG, Hansky J, Eaves ER, et al.: Influence of cigarette smoking on healing and relapse in duodenal ulcer disease. *Gastroenterology* 1983, 85:871.
7. Sontag S, Graham DY, Belsita A, et al.: Cimetidine, cigarette smoking, and recurrence of duodenal ulcer. *New England Journal of Medicine* 1984, 311:689–693.
8. Heatley NG: Some experiments on partially purified gastro-intestinal muco-substance. *Gastroenterology* 1959, 37:304–312.
9. Ganstam SO, Jonson C, Fandriks L, Holm L, Flemstron G: Effects of cigarette smoke and nicotine on duodenal bicarbonate secretion in the rabbit and the rat. *Journal of Clinical Gastroenterology* 1990, 12:519–524.
10. Endoh K, Leung FW: Effects of smoking and nicotine on the gastric mucosa: A review of clinical and experimental evidence. *Gastroenterology* 1994, 107:864–878.
11. Harries AD, Baird A, Rhodes J: Non-smoking: A feature of ulcerative colitis. *British Medical Journal* 1982, 284:706.
12. Motley RJ, Rhodes J, Kay S, Morris TJ: Late presentation of ulcerative colitis in ex-smokers. *International Journal of Colorectal Disease* 1988, 3:171–175.
13. Rudra T, Motley R, Rhodes J: Does smoking improve colitis? *Scandinavian Journal of Gastroenterology* 1989, 24:61–63.
14. Pullan RD, Rhodes J, Ganesh S, Mani V, Morris JS, Williams GT, Newcombe RG, Russell MAH, Feyerabend C, Thomas GAO, Sawe U: Transdermal nicotine for active ulcerative colitis. *New England Journal Medicine* 1994, 330:811–815.
15. Thomas GAO, Rhodes J, Ragunath K, Mani V, Williams GT, Newcombe RG, Russell MAH, Feyerabend C: Transdermal nicotine compared with oral prednisolone for active ulcerative colitis. *European Journal of Gastroenterology and Hepatology* 1996, 8:769–776.
16. Thomas GAO, Rhodes J, Mani V, Williams GT, Newcombe RG, Russell MAGH, Feyerabend C: Transdermal nicotine as maintenance therapy for ulcerative colitis. *New England Journal Medicine* 1995, 332:988–992.
17. Somerville KW, Logan RF, Edmond M, Langman MJ: Smoking and Crohn's disease. *British Medical Journal* 1984, 289:954–956.
18. Rhodes J, Thomas GAO: Smoking good or bad for inflammatory bowel disease? *Gastroenterology* 1994, 106:807–809.
19. Thomas GAO, Davies SV, Rhodes J, Russell MAH, Feyerabend C, Sawe U: Is transdermal nicotine associated with cardiovascular risk? *Journal of the Royal College of Physicians of London* 1995, 29:392–396.
20. Lip GYH: Fibrinogen and cardiovascular disorders. *Quarterly Journal of Medicine* 1995, 88:155–165.

Chapter 16

Adverse Events and Prolonged Use of Nicotine Gum and Patch

DANIEL A. SPYKER, RAYMOND J. ALDERFER,
ROGER A. GOETSCH, A.W. LONGMIRE,
and E. DOUGLAS KRAMER

Nicotine substitution products have been commercially available for a decade. Nicotine gum (2 mg) was first approved by the Food and Drug Administration (FDA) in 1984; the agency approved the 4-mg dose for more highly dependent smokers in 1991. Four transdermal patch systems (5–21 mg/day) were approved in 1991 and 1992. In 1996, nicotine nasal spray was approved as a prescription product, and the gum (2–4 mg) and patch (7–21 mg/day) were approved for over-the-counter sale. In a review of postmarket surveillance, we examined adverse event (AE) reports for the nicotine gum and patch to establish whether possible differences existed in the frequencies of reported dependence on different nicotine delivery systems, with particular attention paid to prolonged use.

We conducted a search of the FDA MedWatch adverse drug event database for reports submitted by patch and gum manufacturers throughout the commercial history of the products. Manufacturers of prescription products are required by law to report all known AEs to the FDA. About 90% of the reports on the nicotine gum and patch came from AE reports originally submitted to the manufacturers. Our search was limited to reports provided by health professionals in the United States because the preponderance of reports received were received from them. We reviewed the epidemiology, total reports, number of prescriptions, and frequency of addiction or dependence (or long-term use) in available AE reports. In our review, we also accounted for patient demography, duration of use, dose, and associated AEs culled from individual case reports of dependence.

Data submission and research methods

Prior to initiation of the MedWatch program in 1993,[1] AE reports were submitted on "form FDA 1639."[2] The "MedWatch form 3500" (FDA 1639) is coded with descriptive terms from a standard dictionary called "COSTART" (coding symbols for thesaurus of adverse drug event terms).[3] Between one and four different COSTART terms are assigned to each report. In conducting the MedWatch database searches, groups of COSTART terms were first chosen as appropriate for the nicotine substitution products. The number of reports with occurrences of one or more of the COSTART terms in each group was then counted (each report could count only once in each group). A report could, however, be counted in more than one COSTART group if it had been assigned more than one associated COSTART term.

We found that 9,574 COSTART terms were associated with the 5,129 AE reports we examined, so the number of COSTART terms used per report averaged about two. For each group and each route, we calculated the number of AE reports, the number in each group per total number of AE reports, and the number in each group per number of new nicotine product prescriptions. The number of new prescriptions for each product was derived from a commercial information service.[4]

As FDA researchers, we had a specific interest in dependence (or long-term use); we reviewed a statistical sampling of reports of dependence on the nicotine gum and patch. Data elements abstracted from the reports included patient demographics, dose of nicotine replacement product, duration of dependence/addiction (long-term use), and success of smoking cessation. We also considered delivery profiles for the gum and patch.

Adverse events

Using COSTART terms, we determined that, overall, there were more than three times the number of AE reports citing the patch as those citing gum. Among cases reported as "serious," the nicotine patch was cited more than four times as often as the gum, and the patch-related AEs were four times more likely to require hospitalization than gum-related AEs. More than five times the number of AE-associated deaths occurred using the patch.

Retail pharmacies dispensed a total of 12.3 million new prescriptions for gum and 11.8 million for the patch. While the number of new gum prescriptions dropped with the introduction of the patch, the 6.7 million patch prescriptions in 1992 is more than threefold the 1.9 million gum prescriptions in 1984 (Fig. 16-1). The total number of reports received by year involving hospitalization, including 56 (4.4%) for gum and 227 (5.9%) for the patch, are shown in Figure 16-2.

A breakdown of the 5,129 reports by COSTART terms permitted a comparison

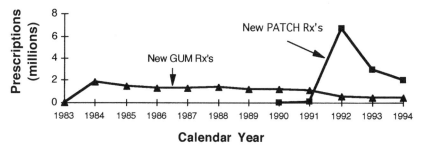

Figure 16-1. New prescriptions by route versus time.

between the AEs reported with gum and patch by percentage of those reported. The categories used to designate specific categories of AE were not standard COSTART Organ System designations, but rather were chosen for this particular study based on their suitability for reviewing nicotine-related AEs.

In terms of site reactions, patch-related AEs made up 29.7% of those reported, with another 24.1% associated with rashes; only 0.23% of the gum AEs were associated with site reactions and 1.17% with rashes. In every other AE category, except for dental (only gum problems were cited for dental), gum was cited significantly less often than the patch. For instance, three times as many gastrointestinal-related events were reported for the patch as for the gum. More than 18 times the number of allergy-related events occurred with patch use than with gum chewing. Nearly five times the number of nervous system–related events occurred with the patch, and patch-related psychiatric events such as insomnia, dream abnormalities, and nervousness were more than 30 times as frequent with the patch as with gum. Finally, an overview of several categories including general and body as a whole, pain, cardiovascular system, musculoskeletal system, and respiratory system showed that the patch was more than eight times as likely to be associated with an AE than the gum.

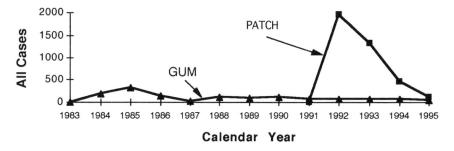

Figure 16-2. Adverse event reports by route (distribution by year of the 5,129 AEs received).

Delivery route pharmacodynamics

The AE patterns differ somewhat between oral and transdermal nicotine delivery, and these differences appear to reflect variations in the local effects of the route of delivery. Most prominently, among the AEs there is approximately 40% reporting of skin irritation with the patch and approximately 23% reporting of oral irritation with gum. Differences in other AE rates may reflect differences in nicotine pharmacodynamics as a function of method and route of administration absorption rate constant, Ka= 5 /hour, time of peak concentration, tpeak = 20 minutes for gum; Ka = 1 /hour, tpeak = 1–3 hours for the patch).

We used a single-compartment linear model to provide an absorption half-life and time of peak concentration. Figure 16-3 shows the blood level profiles for the gum (4 mg) and the best (least squares) fit to a single-compartment linear model. Figure 16-4 shows the blood level profiles for the 21 mg per day patch and the corresponding best (least squares) fit.

Long-term use

While the number of new prescriptions is at best a crude estimate for the number of persons exposed to these products, the rate of dependence and addiction reports is clearly higher for the gum than for the patch. Long-term use of gum has been observed in both actual use and clinical trials, but the exact frequency with which it occurs is unknown. Postmarketing data from adult smokers do not support an association between long-term use and an increase in AEs.

The use of all strengths of gum, and especially the patch, probably overestimates the number of patients starting the therapy. The higher rates of dependence and addiction (principally prolonged use) with the gum may reflect the greater

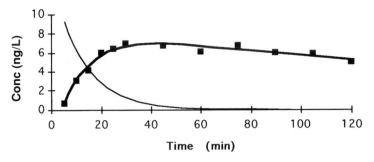

Figure 16-3. Mean blood concentration versus time for Nicotine Polacrilex 4 mg gum (pharmacokinetic solution, 12 observations from 24 patients).

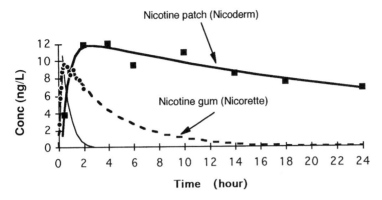

Figure 16-4. Mean blood concentration versus time: 21 mg per day patch (pharmacokinetic solution, nine observations from product labeling).

user involvement with administration and different pharmacokinetics (see Delivery route pharmacodynamics, above).

Limitations of data

The limitations of the use of spontaneous AE reports are well known; they include variable and incomplete reporting, increases in AE reporting over time, some duplication in reports, and lack of causality assessment. Other limitations include occasional assignment of multiple COSTART terms per report numerator; variance of total numbers of reports with product maturity, since manufacturers are required to report AEs more frequently during the first couple of years of marketing[5]; variation in mix of AEs, especially with media attention paid to select ones; and crude estimation of the number of new prescriptions for the number of persons exposed.

The quality of the FDA's Spontaneous Reporting System depends on its reporters. The FDA is concerned about the general safety of all prescription and nonprescription drugs and recommends that any suspected drug-induced illness or injury be reported so that appropriate evaluation and follow up can take place. While drug manufacturers are required to report known AEs, follow-up information is derived primarily from physicians within the United States. In an effort to minimize physician time in reporting AEs, the FDA allows clinicians to contact the agency by telephone and dictate the report (with the FDA transcribing it), fax or mail a copy of a report to the FDA, or contact the FDA via the Internet. The FDA's statistical data have been—and will continue to be—in the hands of health care providers who accurately report AEs associated with nicotine-containing or other drug products. Though much has been learned from existing AE reports, a

clearer picture of nicotine substitution products can only emerge through ongoing, timely, and accurate reporting of AEs by health care providers.

References

1. Kennedy DL, McGinnis T: Monitoring adverse drug reactions: The FDA's new Med-
   Watch program—New guidelines for ADR monitoring. *Pharmacy and Therapeutics*
   1993, 18:833–42.
2. Lee B, Turner W: Food and Drug Administration's adverse drug reaction monitoring
   program. *American Journal of Hospital Pharmacy* 1978, 35:929–932.
3. Food and Drug Administration: *"COSTART" Coding Symbols for* Thesaurus of Adverse Drug Event Terms, *5th ed. 1995.*
4. IMS America: *National Prescription Audit.* IMS America Limited, Plymouth Meeting,
   PA: 1974–1994.
5. Weber JCP: Epidemiology of adverse reactions to nonsteroidal anti-inflammatory
   drugs. In KD Rainsford, GP Velo (eds): *Advances in Inflammation Research,* vol 6.
   New York: Raven Press, 1984, pp 1–7.

Chapter 17

Long-Term
Nicotine Therapy

ROBERT P. MURRAY and KATHLEEN DANIELS

In this volume, there is a considerable review of the literature regarding the safety of nicotine replacement therapy (NRT) from various perspectives. This chapter focuses on the recent experience of more than 3,000 NRT users (Nicorette 2 mg; nicotine polacrilex) in the Lung Health Study.[1] This study provides the single largest source of data on the safety of nicotine medication. In the Lung Health Study, 5,887 volunteer participants were enrolled for 5 years. An intensive smoking cessation and maintenance program, which included the use of NRT, was provided. Over the course of the study, the use of NRT evolved into a relatively long-term treatment with relatively high doses provided for up to 5 years.

The study began in early 1987, with NRT usage guidelines corresponding to the package insert. Recommended use of the gum was 10 or 12 pieces per day. The limit was 30 pieces per day. The original guideline was that NRT was not to be used for more than 6 months. Later, circumstances resulted in modifications to the way in which NRT was dispensed.

As the study progressed, the investigators began to see that participants who used NRT liberally, and for a longer period of time (i.e., exceeding the recommended 6 months), were more successful at quitting smoking than those who used NRT in cautious amounts and/or for shorter time periods. In addition, measures of the study participants' lung functions indicated a high risk for advancing chronic obstructive pulmonary disease (COPD) if they continued smoking.[2] NRT was supplied free of charge to the study population and their support people, so cost factors were not an issue. The study led to the development of a database of adverse events that were carefully documented and collated. This database became larger than that of any previously published NRT safety study and therefore carried significant weight with the investigators as they amended the study's NRT protocol. These factors reinforced the Lung Health Study's decision on the aggressive use of NRT.

Concurrent use of NRT and cigarettes was an additional concern. It was evident that the use of NRT while continuing to smoke was not going to improve the likelihood of stopping smoking. The protocol of the Lung Health Study forbade the dispensing of NRT to those who reported concurrent smoking. In reality, though, the investigators had limited control over the daily behavior of the participants. Participants who reported past concurrent use of cigarettes and NRT were routinely advised not to do so. Those who pledged not to do so in the future were often given a new supply of NRT; some would then use their NRT inappropriately.

Methods

The Lung Health Study enrolled 5,887 men and women between the ages of 35 and 60 years into a study of the prevention of COPD. To be eligible, participants had to have a ratio of forced expiratory volume in 1 second to forced vital capacity of not more than 70% and a forced expiratory volume in 1 second between 55% and 90% of predicted normal. In addition, participants had to be free of major disease. Two-thirds of the Lung Health Study participants were randomized into the special intervention condition, and these ($n = 3,923$) received the smoking cessation intervention including NRT if they chose to use it. These were the participants in the present analysis, which amounts to a nonblinded NRT study. Half of the special intervention participants were assigned to use inhaled ipratropium bromide (Atrovent) in a double-blind procedure. This was not presumed to affect the risk associated with NRT, but inhaled drug assignment was included in a model predicting cardiovascular events. Baseline characteristics of the Lung Health Study sample and the results of the intent-to-treat analysis have been published previously.[3,4]

The group intervention used a multicomponent, biobehavioral approach in which NRT was an important part. Other aspects of the intervention have been described.[5] Participants visited the clinics 12 times in the first 3 months, and their use of NRT was carefully monitored. From 4 months onward, participants who were using NRT attended the clinics every 2 weeks to replenish their supply. NRT was supplied free of charge to participants for the duration of the study and to their support people for the first 6 months.

Smoking status was measured by self-report, carbon monoxide level in expired air, and salivary cotinine concentration. No substantial differences were found among these, but the present analysis relies on biochemically verified smoking status[6]; NRT use was based on self-reports. Hospitalization was based on self-reports, which, in turn, triggered access of a registration record, physician's discharge summary, operative reports, pathology reports, and radiology reports, when permission was given. Records that contained significant mention of cardiovascular, cancer, or respiratory conditions were forwarded to an independent review board of physicians with specialties in these three areas. They also reviewed the forwarded records of all deaths and provided assessments of the primary causes.

Data presented in the figure and tables in this chapter are from visits conducted within 2 months before or after the enrollment anniversary date.

Results

Study participants in special intervention were 62.4% men with a mean age of 48.5 years (SD for men = 7.0, for women = 6.5). Pack-years at enrollment were 43.1 (SD = 20.4) for men and 36.3 (SD = 16.3) for women. A total of 34% of the men reported previous use of NRT compared with 42% of women.

The use of NRT by special intervention participants is described in Figure 17-1. Levels of use are shown for each scheduled clinic visit, as well as number of pieces used per day, separately for exsmokers and smokers. Two-thirds of the participants who had quit smoking used NRT at the beginning of the study, and by the end these had fallen to 15%. About one-third of the participants assigned to quit smoking were unsuccessful, but reported the use of NRT at the outset, and by the end they amounted to 5%. Exsmoking NRT users consumed an average of eight pieces of gum per day at the outset. Over the course of the study, the protocol forbidding extended NRT use began to be enforced more assertively. One result was that users of small amounts of NRT found it easier to quit, and the mean of the remaining users increased to around 10 pieces per day. NRT used by smokers remained at approximately six or seven pieces per day for the duration of the study.

Average salivary cotinine levels (ng/ml) by validated smoking status and self-reported NRT use are listed in Table 17-1.

Smokers of pipes and cigars are classified as smokers in Table 17-1, and those using snuff, chewing tobacco, or nicotine patches are excluded. After the first annual visit, the Lung Health Study measured cotinine on only a subset of self-reported smokers as a cost-saving measure.

Both exsmokers and smokers using NRT appear to have progressively higher cotinine levels over the first 4 years of the study followed by a decrease in year 5. At year 5, the reduction in cotinine levels is likely due to a particular emphasis by the clinics on reduction of NRT use. Smokers not using NRT have essentially constant mean cotinine levels throughout the study. Both exsmokers and smokers

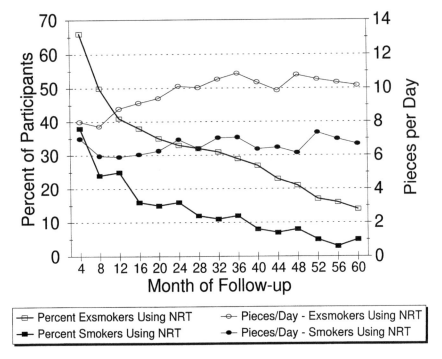

Figure 17-1. Percent and mean amount of reported use of nicotine polacrilex by Special Intervention smokers and ex-smokers.

using NRT appear to achieve mean cotinine levels, particularly in year 4, that exceed the mean cotinine level of smokers not using NRT.

Cardiovascular conditions

There were 188 first hospitalizations and 19 deaths due to cardiovascular events among the participants between the 4-month visit and the 5-year anniversary. Table 17-2 shows the overall rates of hospitalization for cardiovascular events classified by smoking status and NRT use.

Among exsmokers, the rates appear uniformly higher for those not using NRT. Among smokers, the rates for NRT users appear higher in some years, and the rates for NRT nonusers appear higher in others.

Proportional hazards regression was performed to predict fatal and nonfatal cardiovascular events among the 3,325 special intervention participants who had 4-month follow-up records (see Table 17-3).

NRT use had a marginally significant protective effect for cardiovascular events in this sample. Smoking had a significant risk effect. There was an interac-

Table 17-1. Average salivary cotinine levels (ng/ml) for special intervention participants by validated smoking status and self-reported NRT use (standard deviations in parentheses)*

Annual Visit No.	Exsmokers				Smokers†			
	NRT Users (SD)	n	NRT Nonusers (SD)	n	NRT Users (SD)	n	NRT Nonusers (SD)	n
1	217.5 (147.8)	529	2.2 (21.1)	750	291.1 (161.3)	473	298.9 (138.6)	1,374
2	280.8 (223.9)	416	1.2 (7.9)	844	319.0 (187.1)	232	302.5 (156.7)	970
3	314.9 (231.1)	360	1.1 (10.1)	902	325.0 (221.8)	100	301.6 (219.3)	409
4	351.5 (285.5)	262	2.2 (20.8)	981	351.3 (280.5)	51	299.7 (200.7)	374
5	321.3 (278.2)	171	3.5 (31.4)	1,087	314.5 (246.1)	33	311.2 (200.5)	438

*Pipe and cigar smokers or those with missing smoking data were classified as smokers. Any using snuff, chewing tobacco, or nicotine patches (asked at annual visits 4 and 5 only) were excluded. All those with nonmissing NRT and cotinine data are included.

†Note that cotinine was measured only in a subset of smokers after the firs annual visit.

Table 17-2. Hospitalization rates* for cardiovascular conditions among special intervention participants[†] by year in study, use of NRT, and use of cigarettes

Time in Study (Months)	Exsmokers[‡]				Smokers			
	NRT Users	n	NRT Nonusers	n	NRT Users	n	NRT Nonusers	n
4–12	1.27	1,243	6.54	641	0.91	550	4.65	887
12–24	0.53	526	2.85	807	7.07	466	5.67	1,507
24–36	4.38	419	7.34	864	11.76	329	5.62	1,667
36–48	3.72	370	5.78	929	5.12	219	6.02	1,726
48–60	2.29	265	6.44	1,054	9.10	134	6.69	1,748
Overall	2.23		5.78		6.40		5.87	

*Hospitalizations per 100,000 person-days. Includes multiple hospitalizations per person (up to eight) that occurred between the first 4-month visit and the last attended follow-up visit.

[†]n = 3,321 special intervention participants who attended at least one annual visit and for whom complete data for the first 4-month visit were available. n for each interval are the numbers *entering* the interval.

[‡]Categories for smoking and NRT use are determined at the start of each 4-month interval. Missing data were handled as follows: Participants missing smoking information were assumed to be smoking; participants missing NRT information were assumed to be not using NRT.

tion, again marginally significant, between NRT use and log time, suggesting that the protective effect decreased with time. Other control factors in the model were gender, age, and diastolic blood pressure.

A risk effect for the concurrent use of tobacco and NRT would have been expressed as a significant interaction term between smoking and NRT use. Such an interaction was added to the model, but was not significant ($p = 0.63$). A model

Table 17-3. Proportional hazards regression* predicting fatal and nonfatal cardiovascular events among 3,325 special intervention participants

Covariate	Coefficient	SE	RR	95% CI	p
NRT use	− 1.915	1.152	0.15	0.02–1.41	0.10
Current smoker[†]	0.473	0.150	1.61	1.20–2.16	0.002
NRT use by Log time[†‡]	0.286	0.180	—	—	0.11
Gender (Risk = male)	0.926	0.179	2.52	1.78–3.59	< 0.0001
Age (Risk/decade)	0.759	0.115	2.14	1.71–2.68	< 0.0001
Diastolic blood pressure (Risk/ 10 mm Hg)	0.181	0.078	1.20	1.03–1.40	0.02

*Stratified on Lung Health Study clinic.

[†]Entered as a time-dependent covariate. Categories for smoking and NRT use are determined at the start of each 4-month interval. Missing data were handled as follows: Participants missing smoking information were assumed to be smoking; participants missing NRT information were assumed to be not using NRT.

[‡]"Time" is entered as number of days of follow up after the first 4-month visit.

that substituted NRT dose and the interaction of NRT dose with log time led to the same conclusions. Neither NRT dose nor the interaction of NRT dose with log time was significant. To assess the effect of assignment to active versus placebo inhaler groups on cardiovascular risk associated with NRT use, or on the NRT by log time interaction, the analysis in Table 17-3 was repeated including an inhaler assignment term and the appropriate interaction terms. There was no significant interaction between inhaler use and NRT use; neither was there a significant interaction between inhaler use and NRT use and log time.

Peptic ulcers

Special intervention participants who reported a history of peptic ulcer were not eligible to receive NRT from the Lung Health Study unless they received a prescription from their primary care physician. Excluding these participants who reported peptic ulcers at baseline or at the 4-month visit, a proportional hazards regression was used to assess the extent to which NRT may have contributed to the existence of new ulcers. During the 5 years following the 4-month visit, and up to the end of the study, there were 116 self-reported new ulcers. The model is shown in Table 17-4.

NRT, smoking, gender, and age were entered as covariates. NRT was found to have a marginally significant protective effect against peptic ulcers. Further analysis found no effect of NRT dose or of the interaction of either NRT use or NRT dose with log follow-up time on the occurrence of peptic ulcers.

Discussion

Data on hospitalizations have not previously been presented from a study including NRT users and nonusers. The rates of hospitalization reported in this study

Table 17-4. Proportional hazards regression* predicting new cases of peptic ulcer among 3,068 special intervention participants

Covariate	Coefficient	SE	RR	95% CI	p
NRT use[†]	− 0.463	0.250	0.63	0.39–1.03	0.06
Current smoker[†]	− 0.084	0.192	0.92	0.63–1.34	0.66
Gender (Risk = male)	0.247	0.200	1.28	0.87–1.90	< 0.22
Age (Risk/decade)	0.287	0.140	1.33	1.01–1.75	< 0.04

*Stratified on Lung Health Study clinic.

[†]Entered as a time-dependent covariate. Categories for smoking and NRT use are determined at the start of each 4-month interval. Missing data were handled as follows: Participants missing smoking information were assumed to be smoking; participants missing NRT information were assumed to be not using NRT; participants missing data on ulcers were assumed to not have ulcers.

were low, considering the population of heavy smokers with evidence of early COPD. This was interpreted as a healthy volunteer effect, because participants were required to have no significant comorbidities at baseline.

There seemed to be a protective effect of NRT that dissipated over time, both in cardiovascular disease and peptic ulcers. This was not statistically significant in either case. There may have been a protective effect whereby smoking cessation, a physiologically stressful event, was softened in its impact by the use of NRT. Participants with borderline disease and quitting smoking without NRT may have been more likely to experience events. The testing of such a hypothesis was beyond the capacity of this study.

There was no evidence of a relationship between dose of NRT and either cardiovascular disease or peptic ulcers. Lung Health Study participants were on average heavy users of NRT. The dose of NRT varied widely, but mean salivary cotinine levels in NRT-using exsmokers exceeded mean cotinine levels in cigarette smokers (not using NRT) by year 4 in the study. This result was unexpected in the context of what had been reported previously.[7,8]

Although users of NRT were instructed not to smoke, about 16.5% of the special intervention participants reported doing so at their first 4-month clinic visit. Clearly, the efficacy of NRT as a part of the process of quitting smoking was nullified in those who smoked and used NRT concomitantly. It has also been suggested that concomitant use is dangerous to health. Although this study was not designed to test this in detail, no evidence of it was found.

Based on an analysis of hospitalization data in relation to NRT use, there was no evidence of serious side effects; therefore, we conclude that NRT is safe as used in the Lung Health Study.

Epilogue

It has been suggested that the protective effect of NRT in these analyses may be a product of the study design. Absence of NRT use is correlated with smoking. The suggestion was that with smoking status in the model, adjustments are made for something that is strongly correlated with outcome. A model should be considered without adjusting for smoking. This analysis is shown in Table 17-5.

In Table 17-5, NRT use is slightly more protective than it is in Table 17-3. Comparing the -2 log likelihood for the with- and without-smoking status models, the difference is 10.3, which under a χ^2 distribution with 1 df indicates that adding smoking status results in a better model. Because the true outcome variable is fatal/nonfatal cardiovascular disease, the best model is probably the original one, which adjusts for smoking status as a major confounder and thus gives a more accurate estimate of the effects of NRT.

In the case of peptic ulcer, the omission of smoking status results in a model

Table 17-5. Proportional hazards regression* predicting fatal and nonfatal cardiovascular events among 3,325 special intervention participants, excluding smoking status as a covariate

Covariate	Coefficient	SE	RR	95% CI	p
NRT use[†]	− 2.019	1.149	0.13	0.01–1.26	0.08
NRT use by log time[†,‡]	0.284	0.179			0.11
Gender (Risk = male)	0.909	0.179	2.48	1.75–3.53	< 0.0001
Age (Risk/decade)	0.748	0.115	2.11	1.69–2.64	< 0.0001
Diastolic blood pressure (Risk/10 mm Hg)	0.174	0.079	1.19	1.02–1.39	0.03

*Stratified on Lung Health Study clinic.

[†]Entered as a time-dependent covariate. Categories for smoking and NRT use are determined at the start of each 4-month interval. Missing data were handled as follows: Participants missing smoking information were assumed to be smoking; participants missing NRT information were assumed to be not using NRT.

[‡]"Time" is entered as number of days of follow up after the first 4-month visit.

where NRT is still protective. The difference between the models, however, is not significant.

Acknowledgments

Much of the material in this chapter has been previously published in *Chest* and is reproduced here with permission. This study was supported by contract N01-HR-46002 from the Division of Lung Diseases of the National Heart, Lung, and Blood Institute. Boehringer Ingelheim Pharmaceuticals, Marion Merrell Dow, and Merrell Dow Pharmaceuticals (Canada) contributed drugs used in the study.

References

1. Murray RP, et al.: Safety of nicotine polacrilex gum used by 3,094 participants in the Lung Health Study. *Chest* 1996, 109:438–445.
2. Tang JL, et al.: How effective is nicotine replacement therapy in helping people to stop smoking? *British Medical Journal* 1994, 308:21–26.
3. Buist AS, et al.: Chronic obstructive pulmonary disease early intervention trial (Lung Health Study): Baseline characteristics of randomized participants. *Chest* 1993, 103: 1863–1872.
4. Anthonisen NR, et al.: Effects of smoking intervention and the use of an inhaled anticholinergic bronchodilator on the rate of decline of FEV_1: The Lung Health Study. *Journal of the American Medical Association* 1994, 272:1497–1505.
5. O'Hara P, et al.: Design and results of the initial intervention program for the Lung Health Study. *Preventive Medicine* 1993, 22:304–315.
6. Murray RP, et al.: Error in smoking measures: Effects of intervention on relations of cotinine and carbon monoxide to self-reported smoking. *American Journal of Public Health* 1993, 83:1251–1257.

7. Russell MAH: Nicotine replacement: The role of blood nicotine levels, their rate of change, and nicotine tolerance. In Pomerleau OF, Pomerleau CS (eds): *Nicotine Replacement: A Critical Evaluation.* New York: Alan R Liss, 1988, pp 63–94.

8. Tønnesen P: Dose and nicotine dependence as determinants of nicotine gum efficacy. In Pomerleau OF, Pomerleau CS (eds): *Nicotine Replacement: A Critical Evaluation.* New York: Alan R Liss, 1988, pp 129–144.

Part VI

Conclusion

This volume provides a comprehensive review of nicotine safety and toxicity. Although the focus of this volume is not tobacco, it should be emphasized that all of the evidence indicates that nicotine administered as a medication is always safer than that obtained by cigarette smoking. Cigarette smoke contains a variety of carcinogens, oxidants, irritants, and other injurious chemicals that are responsible for most of the harmful effects of tobacco use.

The main health concerns related to nicotine, per se, have been cardiovascular disease, cancer, reproductive disturbances, behavioral toxicity, and gastrointestinal disease. This chapter reviews the main conclusions of authors regarding the toxicity of nicotine in these various areas.

Chapter 18

Summary:
Risks and Benefits of Nicotine

NEAL L. BENOWITZ

General considerations

Before considering specific disease conditions, it is essential to understand that the safety of nicotine depends very much on the dose, pattern, and duration of exposure (see Chapter 2) There are many data on the safety and toxicity of nicotine products administered for several months to aid smoking cessation, showing that the risks of such therapy are minimal. The risk of long-term therapy, such as might be entertained if treating chronic medical conditions, is as yet unknown. The rapidity of nicotine dosing is important in that rapid dosing results in much higher arterial concentrations and high concentrations at the sites of nicotine effects, including the brain and the heart. These high concentrations may have implications for both cardiovascular toxicity and behavioral toxicity. There is also evidence that the dose–response relationship for cardiovascular effects of nicotine is relatively flat such that low doses of nicotine may have as much cardiovascular impact as high doses of nicotine. This would seem to offer some reassurance with respect to adverse cardiovascular effects of higher dose nicotine, particularly the situation of combined nicotine administration and cigarette smoking. The dose–response relationship for other pharmacological effects, however, remains to be characterized.

Cardiovascular disease

The main observations relating nicotine to cardiovascular disease are as follows. Nicotine exerts its most important cardiovasular effects by activating the sympathetic nervous system, resulting in an increase in heart rate, blood pressure, and cardiac contractility, thereby increasing myocardial oxygen consumption and demand for blood flow (see Chapters 1 and 3). Nicotine may also limit coronary blood flow by constricting coronary arteries, an effect that is more prominent in individuals with underlying coronary atherosclerosis. Other important cardiovascular toxins in cigarette smoke include carbon monoxide, which reduces oxygen delivery to the heart, and oxidant gases, which may be responsible for endothelial dysfunction and platelet activation.[1] Effects on endothelial function and platelets, mediated by oxidant gases, may be responsible for the thrombosis and/or coronary vasoconstriction that further restricts blood flow to the heart. Nicotine per se, at least when administered transdermally, does not seem to activate platelets and probably does not contribute to thrombosis.

Data on the cardiovascular effects of nicotine in animals raise some concerns about toxicity with long-term exposure (see Chapter 3). Some, but not all, studies find that nicotine accelerates the development of atherosclerosis. These studies have been performed primarily in animals on diets that have induced marked hypercholesterolemia and in the context of high-dose nicotine therapy. One biological basis for accelerated atherosclerosis might be nicotine-mediated increases in low-density lipoprotein cholesterol and reduced high-density lipoprotein cholesterol, which have been observed in rabbits and monkeys. There is some evidence from cell culture and in vivo animal studies that nicotine is toxic to endothelial cells. Calcium may contribute to nicotine-induced atherosclerosis, as suggested by the interaction between nicotine and vitamin D to produce atherosclerosis in rabbits. Overall, studies in animals suggest that chronic nicotine exposure in combination with hypercholesterolemia could accelerate atherogenesis.

Studies of the effects of smokeless tobacco use provide further evidence regarding the cardiovascular safety of nicotine (see Chapter 4). Smokeless tobacco users experience the same levels of nicotine in the body as cigarette smokers, but are not exposed to tar, carbon monoxide, and combustion gases. There is a significant pharmacokinetic difference with respect to rate of absorption such that cigarette smoking produces much higher transient arterial blood concentrations than does smokeless tobacco, which must be kept in mind as a caveat in comparing nicotine exposures from the two routes. Snuff use does result in acute cardiovascular effects similar to those with cigarette smoking, that is, an increase in heart rate and blood pressure. Cigarette smoking has been shown to affect platelet activation, as evidenced by increased thromboxane A_2 metabolite excretion and impaired endothelial function, primarily by reducing the release of nitric oxide, which has antiplatelet activity and is a vasodilator. None of the effects on thromboxane A_2 or nitric oxide is seen with snuff users, suggesting that the effect of smoking on these physiological functions is not mediated by nicotine. However, results from epidemiological studies of cardiovascular disease in snuff users are conflicting. One case–control study found no increased risk of myocardial infarction in snuff users.[2] Another cohort study did report an increased risk.[3] The reason for the discrepancies between these two studies is unclear, and further work along this line is needed.

Clinical trials of nicotine medication in patients with coronary artery disease provide another important source of information (see Chapter 5). Two controlled clinical trials of transdermal nicotine to aid smoking cessation in patients with documented cardiovascular disease have found no evidence that nicotine is injurious.[4,5] Importantly, many of the subjects of these studies have continued to smoke while using transdermal nicotine, resulting in plasma nicotine levels that might have been higher than those seen with smoking alone. A study examining quantitative thallium perfusion defect size in smokers with coronary heart disease who were prescribed nicotine patches to aid smoking cessation was conducted.[6] When these subjects were using 21-mg nicotine patches, their blood levels of nicotine and cotinine were twice those seen with smoking alone. Expired carbon monoxide levels were reduced by about 50% because they smoked fewer cigarettes. The total and reversible thallium perfusion sizes were significantly reduced during patch use, despite the high nicotine levels. This study suggests that it is components of cigarette smoke other than nicotine that are responsible for acute ischemia. Finally, the large Health Lung Study in patients with chronic obstructive lung disease found no increase of cardiovascular disease in smokers using nicotine gum for as long as 5 years (see Chapter 17). Thus, all of the clinical trials to date support the idea that nicotine is not a significant risk factor for cardiovascular events even in patients with coronary heart disease.

The data on nicotine and cardiovascular disease may be synthesized by level of probability of concern based on potential mechanisms, experimental and clinical evidence, and concerns for specific cardiovascular diseases. Potential mechanisms of adverse effects are summarized in Table 18-1. The hemodynamic effects of nicotine definitely could contribute to acute cardiovascular events. The experimental data in animals suggest some concern with long-term exposure. The clinical data are reassuring, showing that transdermal nicotine does not increase the risk of acute cardiovascular events. The probabilities of risk with nicotine therapy with respect to particular cardiovascular diseases are shown in Table 18-2. Overall, it can be stated with a high degree of certainty that, while nicotine has some potential for acutely aggravating cardiovascular disease, nicotine is much less hazardous than cigarette smoking, which exposes individuals to nicotine as well as to many other potential cardiovasular toxins. One area that has not been adequately researched is the effect of nicotine on patients with unstable cardiovascular problems such as unstable angina or acute myocardial infarction.

Table 18-1. Possible mechanisms of cardiovascular toxicity of nicotine

Mechanism	Probability
Hemodynamic effects	Definite
Coronary vasoconstriction	Definite
Adverse serum lipid effects	Possible
Endothelial cell toxicity	Possible
Accelerated atherosclerosis	Possible, especially in association with other risk factors
Thrombosis	Doubtful
Arrhythmias	Possible, especially atrial

Cancer

Because of the strong causal link between tobacco use and cancer, there has been concern as to whether nicotine contributes to cancer. Many carcinogens act via chemically reactive metabolic intermediates that covalently bind to macromolecules such as DNA. As reviewed in Chapter 6, nicotine has been shown to be metabolized to nicotine iminium ion, which is then normally oxidized to cotinine. Nicotine iminium ion is highly reactive and can covalently bind to microsomal proteins. Likewise, nicotine may be metabolized to β-nicotyrine, another compound that can be metabolized to reactive intermediates. Thus, studies of the chemistry of nicotine indicate that reactive intermediates and covalent binding of endogenous biomolecules can occur, although the significance of these observations to human disease is unclear.

Nitrosamines are believed to contribute to tobacco-related cancer (see Chapter 7). Nicotine and related alkaloids can be nitrosated to form potentially carcinogenic tobacco-specific nitrosamines. Tobacco-specific nitrosamines are found in tobacco itself, resulting from the reaction of nitrite and alkaloids in the

Table 18-2. Contribution of nicotine to various cardiovascular disease states

Disease	Probability
Accelerated atherosclerosis	Possible
Acute myocardial infarction	Possible
Unstable angina	Possible
Sudden death	Possible
Aggravation of stable angina	Possible
Peripheral arterial occlusive disease	Possible
Reocclusion of bypass graft or restenosis after angioplasty	Doubtful
Stroke	Possible

cigarette tobacco curing process. Of concern with respect to the toxicity of nicotine per se is whether nitrosamine formation can occur in the human body.

Nitrosamines can be formed in the gastrointestinal tract after oral administration of secondary amines and nitrites. Human exposure to nitrites occurs through the diet, and nicotine enters the gastrointestinal tract both by swallowing products such as the nicotine in gum, inhaler, or nasal spray and by diffusion from the bloodstream and ionic trapping by the acidic gastric fluid. Nitrosation of nicotine has not been observed in simulated human saliva or gastric juice, but has been observed after intragastric administration of nicotine and nitrite in rats. Studies of urinary concentrations of nitrosamines in humans exposed to nicotine are underway. It is likely that some nitrosation occurs, but the unresolved question is whether the amount of nicotine-derived nitrosamines is sufficient to contribute to cancer.

Another mechanism by which nicotine could contribute to cancer is via stimulation of nicotinic cholinergic receptors that regulate release of lung tumor growth factors (see Chapter 8). Nicotine can induce a proliferative response of neoplastic pulmonary neuroendocrine cells. Of interest, this response was seen only at high carbon dioxide levels. High carbon dioxide levels are seen in humans with severe chronic obstructive lung disease, which is known to be a risk factor for the development of smoking-induced lung cancer. Conversely, desensitization of nicotinic cholinergic receptors occurs with chronic nicotine exposure, which could result in suppression of tumor growth. The relevance of these studies to human lung cancer is unclear as yet.

Nicotine could contribute to cancer by several mechanisms. Clearly, the risk of nicotine-related cancer, if any, is small or insignificant in tobacco users who are exposed to high concentrations of many carcinogens. There remains a possibility that long-term exposure to nicotine could contribute to cancer, although it appears, at present, that that risk is small. Nicotine has not been shown to be carcinogenic in animals. More research is needed to quantitate the generation of nicotine-derived nitrosamines in humans. Long-term epidemiological studies of cancer in Swedish snuff users might be revealing. To date, there is no evidence of an increased risk of cancer among Swedish snuff users, whose snuff is relatively low in nitrosamine content. In contrast, there is a relationship between snuff use and oral cancer in the United States, because U.S. snuff contains much higher levels of nitrosamines.[7]

Reproductive toxicity of nicotine

Cigarette smoking during pregnancy results in an increased risk of spontaneous abortion, abruptio placenta, and low birth weight. There is also concern about neonatal neurotoxicity and an increased risk of sudden infant death syndrome (SIDS). A role of nicotine in some or all of these disorders is suspected, but not proven. The toxicity of nicotine is of particular concern in that there are clear benefits in the use of nicotine replacement therapy as an adjunct to smoking cessation during pregnancy.

Chapter 11 reviews nicotine and obstetrical complications. A teratogenic effect of nicotine has been shown with high-dose nicotine administration in animals and could contribute to the increased risk of spontaneous abortion in smokers. Growth restriction is seen in fetuses of smokers who continued to smoke beyond week 16 of pregnancy. In animals, nicotine results in lower birth weight, an effect that most likely is related to reduction of placental blood flow.

Chapter 9 describes how nicotine might produce fetal neurotoxicity, acting on nicotinic cholinergic receptors that control neuronal cell differentiation. Premature activation of nicotinic cholinergic receptors in the early stage of fetal development may result in arrested neural cell replication and impaired neural cell development in animals. Similar effects are seen on adrenal chromaffin cells, which are responsible for releasing catecholamines in response to stress, including hypoxemia. Neurotoxicity that results from nicotine exposure could result in impaired behavioral development in young children of smokers and could explain, at least in part, the association between maternal cigarette smoking and greater risk of SIDS. Chapter 10 reviews the effects of maternal smoking on infant development and describes ways in which neonatal exposure to nicotine during and after pregnancy can be quantitated.

Based on available data, there is a probable relationship between nicotine and spontaneous abortion, low birth weight, and neonatal neurotoxicity. There is a possible relationship between nicotine and SIDS. The possibility that neonatal exposure to nicotine might result in a greater risk for the development of nicotine dependence in offspring has also been raised, although to date there is no evidence to support this concept.

While nicotine therapy during pregnancy is potentially harmful or hazardous, it is likely that nicotine therapy is less hazardous than cigarette smoking, which exposes the mother and fetus to both nicotine and a myriad of other toxins. The benefits of successful smoking cessation with the use of nicotine replacement therapies clearly outweigh the risks of nicotine per se. However, it seems prudent not to expose the fetus to more nicotine than it would have been exposed to from cigarette smoking. As discussed in Chapter 10, it is possible to measure cotinine levels in a pregnant woman prior to cessation therapy and then to adjust the nicotine dose so that it does not exceed baseline cotinine levels.

Several important research questions regarding nicotine and pregnancy need to be addressed. It is important to ascertain if there is a critical time period of exposure that increases the risk of obstetrical or fetal toxicity. Likewise, it is important to know whether there is a dose threshold of toxicity. A pharmacokinetic model for the human mother and fetus would allow modeling of nicotine exposure from cigarette smoking and from various types of nicotine replacement therapy. Such a model would be extemely useful in selecting the best type of, and optimal dosing schedule for, nicotine replacement therapy. Finally, there is a need for biomarkers of neural development in neonates to better assess the potential toxic effects of nicotine.

Behavioral toxicity

Because nicotine is responsible for physical dependence and addiction with the use of tobacco, it is of obvious concern that these types of problems might occur with the use of pure nicotine products. Chapter 12 addresses the abuse liability of nicotine, pointing out the prime importance of pharmacokinetic factors. The rapidity of absorption and speed of onset are extremely important in determining the abuse liability of a nicotine product. The more rapid the absorption, the more likely it is that a drug will be abusable, both because of the development of high arterial and, consequently, brain concentrations and the possibility for rapid reinforcement after dosing and titration of effect. Thus, abuse liability is greatest with cigarette smoking, with decreasing abuse liability for nicotine nasal spray, nicotine gum, and nicotine patches, in that order.

Chapter 13 focuses on the acute behavioral effects of nicotine and physical dependence and withdrawal as potential sources of behavioral toxicity. Acute nicotine exposure can impair performance and impede learning of certain tasks. These effects tend to be most pronounced after the first exposure, with substantial development of tolerance developing over time. Thus, it appears that the use of nicotine products in individuals who are tolerant is not likely to be associated with acute behavioral toxicity. Conversely, however, once a person is tolerant, withdrawal symptoms may develop during abstention from nicotine consumption, which may impair concentration, vigilance, and task performance. Another potential behavioral toxicity includes sleep disturbances, which have been mentioned in the postmarketing surveillance studies.

Chapter 14 examines the clinical evidence for dependence and abuse of nicotine medications. A small proportion of former smokers continue to use nicotine gum and nicotine nasal spray for prolonged periods of time. Whether prolonged use of nicotine in this context represents dependence or whether it represents the use to prevent relapse to cigarette smoking is unclear. Long-term patch use has not been a problem, which is consistent with its slow absorption characteristics and minimal acute psychoactivity.

Clearly, there are potential behavioral toxicities of nicotine products that need to be considered in a risk–benefit analysis examining its use for medical diseases. Some unanswered research questions include the likelihood of developing dependence on nicotine in "never smokers" treated with nicotine. We need to better understand the reasons for long-term use of nicotine gum and nicotine nasal spray. Further research is also needed to address the dependence potential for the use of nicotine medications in individuals who have been exsmokers for some time.

Other types of behavioral toxicity that have been of concern for over-the-counter nicotine include the use of nicotine for body weight control and for performance enhancement. This appears not to have been a problem based on early postmarketing surveillance data. Abuse liability testing in particularly vulnerable populations, such as drug abusers and people with affective disorders, is needed. Finally, there is concern about whether the free availability of nicotine products will result in some people continuing tobacco use by virtue of their being able to use nicotine products when they are restricted from smoking, such as in the workplace, rather than stopping smoking altogether.

Gastrointestinal toxicity

Gastrointestinal and metabolic effects of nicotine are of interest both for potential therapeutic utility and for examination of toxicity. As reviewed in Chapter 15, reduction of body weight is a well-established concomitant of cigarette smoking, an effect medicated by actions of nicotine to increase metabolic rate and to suppress appetite. Nicotine ameliorates ulcerative colitis, which is the first medical disorder for which controlled clinical trials of nicotine have been performed. On the other hand, there is evidence that nicotine aggravates gastroesophageal reflux, an effect documented in humans using transdermal nicotine. Nicotine could contribute to duodenal ulceration by decreasing bicarbonate secretion, an effect that may be related to depression of prostaglandin synthesis. However, the results of the Lung Health Study, reviewed in Chapter 17, do not support a role for nicotine in causing peptic disease. The Lung Health found no evidence that nicotine gum use for several years increased the risk of peptic ulcer disease, but rather that gum use had a borderline protective effect. Postmarketing surveillance data likewise found little evidence of serious gastrointestinal toxicity with the use of nicotine products (see Chapter 14).

Gastrointestinal side effects due to nicotine appear to be minor, with the possible exception of gastroesophageal reflux. Gastroesophageal reflux symptoms might be ameliorated by discontinuing the use of nicotine products at night, when reflux symptoms tend to be most severe.

Risks versus benefits of nicotine as a medication

Nicotine as a medication for the treatment of diseases other than smoking cessation shows considerable promise. Diseases for which there are data suggesting benefits to humans include ulcerative colitis and Tourette syndrome.[8] Short-term improvement in cognitive function has been shown after nicotine administration in patients with Alzheimer's disease as well. Data on the epidemiology of cigarette smoking and depression, as well as current understanding of neurochemical actions of nicotine, suggest that depression might benefit from nicotine treatment. Pharmacological considerations and anecdotal clinical reports also indicate that nicotine should be tested in attention deficit disorder, Parkinson's disease, and possibly obesity. The development of nicotine as a medication for these diseases is in a very early stage. The only disease for which controlled clinical trials have been conducted is ulcerative colitis.

While nicotine is a potential toxin, it appears to be well tolerated during weeks and months of nicotine medication therapy without evidence of serious adverse health effects. (See Chapters 16 and 17). Compared with cigarette smoking, which exposes individuals to carbon monoxide and many other combustion products, as well as nicotine, replacement therapy is much less hazardous. Because treatment with nicotine medication can promote smoking cessation, and smoking cessation produces tremendous health benefits, nicotine replacement therapy appears to have a positive benefit/risk ratio for any smoker who cannot quit smoking without nicotine therapy.

Some individuals may stop smoking using nicotine therapy but relapse when they stop the nicotine treatment. For such individuals, the safety of long-term nicotine maintenance therapy has to be considered. Because exposure to nicotine during nicotine replacement therapy is generally no greater than during cigarette smoking, and because there is less exposure to other tobacco toxins, the benefits of nicotine maintenance therapy almost certainly outweighs the risks.

The risks and benefits of long-term nicotine use in nonsmokers being treated for medical diseases is less clear. For intermittent or short-term therapy, such as 3–6-month treatment for control of symptoms of ulcerative colitis, nicotine seems quite safe. The risk/benefit ratio of the use of nicotine for many years, as might be the case in treating depression or attention deficit disorder, remains to be determined. Any analysis of risks and benefits will depend strongly on the magnitude of the beneficial effects of nicotine for particular disorders, which are not yet fully understood.

Acknowledgments

The contributions of the many participants of the Safety and Toxicity of Nicotine Symposium held in Brazelton, Georgia, in November 1996 to the final formation of risks and benefits expressed in this chapter are gratefully acknowledged.

References

1. Benowitz NL, Gourlay SG: Cardiovascular Toxicity of Nicotine: Implications for Nicotine Replacement Therapy. *Journal of the American College of Cardiology* 1997, 29: 1422–1431.

2. Huhtasaari F, Asplund K, Stegmayr B, Wester PO: Tobacco and myocardial infarction: Is snuff less dangerous than cigarettes? *British Medical Journal* 1992, 305:1252–1256.

3. Bolinder G, Alfredsson L, Englund A, de Faire U: Smokeless tobacco use and increased cardiovascular mortality among Swedish construction workers. *American Journal of Public Health* 1994, 84:399–404.

4. Working Group for the Study of Transdermal Nicotine in Patients with Coronary Artery Disease: Nicotine replacement therapy for patients with coronary artery disease. *Archives of Internal Medicine* 1994, 154:989–995.

5. Joseph AM, Norman SM, Ferry LH, Prochazka AV, Westman EC, Steele BG, Sherman SE, Cleveland M, Antonnucio DO, Hartman N, McGovern, PE: The Safety of Transdermal Nicotine as an Aid to Smoking Cessation in Patients with Cardiac Disease. *New England Journal of Medicine,* 1996, 335: 1792–1798.

6. Mahmarian JJ, Moye LA, Nasser GA, Nagueh SF, Bloom MF, Benowitz NL, Verani MS, Byrd WG, Pratt CM: Nicotine patch therapy in smoking cessation reduces the extent of execise-induced myocardial ischemia. *Journal of the American College of Cardiology* 1997, 30:125–130.

7. Winn DJ, Blot WJ, Shy CM, Pickole LW, Toledo A, Fraumeni JF: Snuff dipping and oral cancer among women in the southern United States. *New England Journal of Medicine* 1981, 305:745–749.

8. Benowitz NL: Pharmacology of nicotine: Addiction and therapeutics. *Annual Review of Pharmacology and Toxicology* 1996, 36:597–613.

INDEX

.